# A History of Developmental and Behavioral Pediatrics at the University of Rochester

# A History of Developmental and Behavioral Pediatrics at the University of Rochester

## 1947–2019

Philip W. Davidson and
Susan L. Hyman

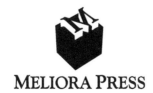

## MELIORA PRESS

An imprint of the University of Rochester Press

First published 2021

Meliora Press is an imprint of the
University of Rochester Press
668 Mt. Hope Avenue, Rochester, NY 14620, USA
and Boydell & Brewer Limited
PO Box 9, Woodbridge, Suffolk IP12 3DF, UK
www.boydellandbrewer.com

ISBN-13: 978-1-64825-019-4

Cataloging-in-Publication data available from the Library of Congress

This publication is printed on acid-free paper.

Printed in the United States of America.

# DEDICATION

Margaret "Peg" Sheehan has been an inspiration since she came to our clinic for children with developmental needs when she was 12 years old. She is now 56 years old. Her multiple disabilities have not affected her good humor, love of her family and friends, and her persistence and determination. She has taught us a great deal about life. But most of all, she has inspired those who crossed her path. To us, she represents all that is good in life, despite obstacles that may intervene. That is why we dedicate this history to her.

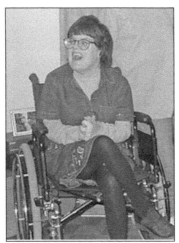

Figure D.1. Margaret "Peg" Sheehan. Photo from family and reproduced with permission.

# CONTENTS

*Contents*

# FOREWORD

Elizabeth R. McAnarney, MD
Distinguished University Professor
Chair Emerita, Department of Pediatrics
University of Rochester
Rochester, NY

This story is about sustained growth leading to change. Growth that promotes and guides change is underpinned by inspiration, innovation, effects on the human condition, and personal and professional commitment." This quote is from the final paragraphs of this remarkable volume, "A History of Developmental and Behavioral Pediatrics at the University of Rochester: 1947–2019." Having been witness to the sustained growth of outstanding developmental and behavioral pediatric programs in the University of Rochester's Department of Pediatrics and allied departments since the late 1960s, I can attest to the fact that the recounting of the historical context within which the programs developed both within the country and within the local environment are portrayed accurately and eloquently. This book is a meticulous chronicling of how the external culture moved from institutionalization, almost warehousing of persons who had intellectual and developmental disabilities, to gradual inclusion in community settings.

These changes demanded visionary leadership to develop new programs to assure that the individuals who had intellectual and developmental disabilities and their families were not placed at undue risk during challenging transitions. New services included the development of safe living environments for persons moving from institutional care to community settings; training of ambulatory interdisciplinary teams of providers; health care, both in a hospital and in the community; education; social services; home services; and integration across services within given programs and between institutions located throughout communities. As the reader will appreciate after reading this history, indeed the leaders of the Rochester program were very much up to this challenging task and skillfully wove together many moving parts in order, over time, to develop an integrated clinical, education, and research effort.

The continuity of leadership of the University of Rochester's Developmental and Behavioral Pediatrics efforts over seven decades and the evolution of the entire program are detailed with great accuracy. The recognition of many members of the team by the authors, including photographs of these individuals, is a highlight that reminds the reader of the many persons and skills needed to even begin to address the complexity of the care of persons who have intellectual disabilities. These persons were charged with the task of developing the various projects and were often under great pressure to jumpstart services; indeed, they did so skillfully. For those such as I who had the privilege of observing the growth of this program, this history reignites the challenges and joys of its development.

Initially, clinicians led the program and were dedicated to assuring that excellent services were available. The thirty years of the programs under Dr. Philip W. Davidson's command have been extended continuously until the present. At the time that Dr. Davidson joined the nascent clinical programs, services and supports for children and adults with intellectual and developmental disabilities were limited but did address consumer and family needs to the best of our abilities at the time. As noted, the then-chairs of the University of Rochester's Department of Pediatrics, Dr. William L. Bradford and Dr. Robert J. Haggerty, defined pediatrics broadly and recognized the high priority on community liaisons with practicing pediatricians, schools, Monroe County Department of Health, and other agencies and hospitals serving people with special needs. At that time, there were few psychologists who were full-time members of the faculty in the clinical departments at medical centers. Dr. Davidson's special skill and comfort in medical settings and the ease with which he worked with colleagues from many disciplines, both within the medical center and within the community, were remarkable. In addition to his ability to relate comfortably with colleagues from multiple backgrounds, his and his colleagues' ingenuity at developing new efforts when funding became available (for example, foreseeing the increase in the number of people who are diagnosed with autism spectrum disorders, children who had multiple and complex diagnoses, and the needs of people with disabilities reaching older age, among others) were stellar. As I read the volume, I could not help but think of several concepts: ingenuity, energy, creativity, flexibility, good will, bravery, persistence, and courage.

Dr. Davidson's coauthor and now division director, Dr. Susan Hyman, carried on Dr. Davidson's vision with similar energy and creativity and has deftly carried the program ever further into the mainstream of our medical center's strategic plan. Major advances in the education and research missions, participation in departmental fund-raising targeted for special projects, and new larger plans for the entire effort all augers well for the population being served.

The narrative describes how over a very long period, key grants and contracts were acquired that form the backbone of any University Center devoted to people with IDD. As early as the late 1950s, attempts were made to define a comprehensive center of excellence that included research, education, service, and community involvement. These included a University Center of Excellence in IDD (UCEDD), a Leadership Education in Neurodevelopmental and Related Disorders (LEND), both of which are in place now. But the third leg of top-tier programs, an Intellectual and Developmental Disabilities Research Center (IDDRC) proved elusive. Just as this book was going to press, the University was notified that its application for an IDDRC had been funded. As Drs. Davidson and Hyman describe, this puts URMC in a very small and elite group of universities. The IDDRC, based in the Del Monte Institute for Neuroscience, is poised to partner with Pediatrics to build something special in Rochester.

The challenges experienced by these leaders and colleagues and in all programs still exist as we look to the future. As noted, people with intellectual and developmental disabilities, largely as a result of earlier success, are living longer and will need new, creative approaches to assure their well-being. Funding of health care in general for individuals and health care institutions, educational programs, supports and services for people with disabilities are constantly under duress and these challenges will only increase over time as the persons who have intellectual and developmental disabilities become a larger part of society as a whole. Competition for funding for every level of research and education endeavors is relentless. It will take continued creativity, energy, and good will to assure that every individual whom we serve can reach his or her potential.

Monroe County/Rochester, New York over the years has been a creative community committed to developing services and supports for persons who are disabled and their families. Over many years, this community is a remarkably generous one. This generosity is reflected not only in charitable contributions, but also in active volunteerism. We will need to continue to nurture many varied sources of revenue including local, state, and federal resources to "create the future" for all persons who have unmet needs for whom we are all responsible.

Let me extend my deepest gratitude and congratulations to my colleagues, Drs. Davidson and Hyman, for assuring that this story about a truly successful effort against all odds on behalf of persons who have disabilities and their families is told and that the individuals who "built the bicycle while riding it," are acknowledged and thanked for their hard work to care for those least able.

*Be brave enough to live life creatively.*
—Alan Alda

# PREFACE

The walls of the University of Rochester Medical Center are covered with plaques, portraits, and photographs placed as tributes to former faculty members, division chiefs, chairs, and deans. Every day of our tenures as faculty members we walk by these remembrances, knowing few if any of them or the many people who worked with them from personal experience. We know very little about these people, some or all of whom played a role in making the Medical Center what it is today.

One of us (Dr. Davidson) is now retired and living in Hilton Head, South Carolina, where he and his wife belong to the World Affairs Council of Hilton Head. This chapter of a nationwide organization sponsors lectures each year for its members. They recently attended a lecture given by Christopher Alexander, a Canadian diplomat and politician. In describing the importance of Quebec to the taxation rules imposed by King George III on the US colonies that eventuated in the Declaration of Independence, he said the taxation legislation "annoyed" George Washington. It's not that interesting, they thought. The only things we know about George Washington are garnered from pictures, movies, and books. They realized they knew nothing about the man himself, his feelings, motivations, and what drove him and others who are our founders to do what they did.

It has been 72 years since intellectual and developmental disabilities (IDD) services were first offered to the community by the Medical Center. Very few people who knew, worked with, or learned from those who started these efforts remain to tell us their feelings, motivations, and what drove them. One of these people is Dr. Neal McNabb. He recently asked Dr. Davidson, "Can I share your manuscript with others in the community?" Dr. Davidson said, "No, it must remain embargoed until published." Dr. McNabb replied, "Hurry up."

We think Dr. McNabb's admonishment was prophetic. We wrote this book to provide readers with some insight into how Rochester's program in IDD began and evolved. But even more important than that, is what moved the founders of this remarkable program to see it through, what vicissitudes of fortune made it possible to move forward, and why they stuck it out.

People with IDD have been a part of society for as long as humankind has existed. For much of world history, people with IDD have been excluded from mainstream society, marginalized, criminalized, and abused (Rafter, 2004). They have been treated as subhuman; during parts of history, society has devised schemes to eliminate them. As recently as the World War II era, people with IDD were sent to concentration camps and gassed. One of us once attended a conference in Vienna that was opened by a past president of Austria. He apologized to the audience, made up largely of researchers working on issues related to aging with IDD, because he said there were no older people with IDD in his country. They had all been exterminated by the Nazis, he said.

It was not until the 1960s that governments in developed nations began to address the shortage of appropriate and necessary services and supports for their citizens with IDD and their families. The need for educational programs to prepare professionals to provide these services and for health care to extend lives is what brought universities into the IDD arena. This book relates the history of how the University of Rochester played a part in addressing these needs. Rooted in 19th and early 20th Century history, the story begins in the late 1940s and continues through the present. Thus, it is a very long story. Why is that? One might say it takes time for good programs to evolve in complex systems such as universities. One might also say that the program at the University of Rochester not only had to develop internal capacity but also link effectively with partners in the community. One might say that good programs require funds to grow. Or one might say that before a program can emerge and blossom, there must be a cultural change from within. All these things are true.

This story is remarkable for several other reasons specific to University of Rochester Medical Center (URMC). First, the University of Rochester's IDD program was developed and flourishes in a private university. In the early years, most university-based programs in IDD were sponsored by public institutions of higher learning. Very few private universities participated. This happened because state mandates for education, service, and research in IDD were connected to state legislative funding streams that in many cases provided a base for federally funded programs to be built. Rochester had no such advantage. Secondly, its development benefited (and continues to benefit) from the wisdom and guidance of institutional leaders in the School of Medicine and Dentistry without whose support, very little would have happened or will continue to happen. Third, like most long stories about how human service programs emerge, there was a combination of hard work, belief in principled growth, and a bit of good old-fashioned timing and luck.

This is the story of the emergence and maturation of a program whose founders (those people whose pictures are displayed on the wall) are nearly all gone. However, the IDD program is still growing and evolving and will do so as long as there are people with IDD and their families in our community who want committed professional partners with vision and compassion to work with them, side by side, to achieve full inclusion in society. This history can serve as a beacon for current and future leaders of the IDD program as it continues to grow in our community. It can also guide program development elsewhere in the University of Rochester and beyond. We have compiled this history as encouragement for the many hundreds of students that have already trained with us and guidance for those yet to come.

This book should stand as a reminder of what it took to get where we are today and that it will require some effort to keep things moving forward. As we do so, we must remember George Santayana's famous aphorism: "Those who cannot remember the past are condemned to repeat it." (Santayana, 1905, p. 284).

Enjoy!

Philip W. Davidson and Susan L. Hyman
March 2021

*"You can't stay in your corner of the Forest waiting for others to come to you. You have to go to them sometimes."*

—A. A. Milne, *Winnie the Pooh*

# Chapter One

# HISTORICAL CONTEXT

*. . . [a] custodial experiment, which was to determine whether the
need existed for such an asylum; whether there are in the county
poorhouses or elsewhere feeble-minded women who need care and
protection to prevent them from multiplying their kind and so
increasing the number of the dependent classes in the State; also,
could they be maintained without undue cost.*

—S.S. Pierson, 1893, from his Historical Address,
delivered at the dedication of the New York Custodial
Asylum for Feeble-Minded Women, at Newark, N.Y.,
June 10, 1890

People with intellectual and developmental disabilities (IDD)
have been a part of our culture and experience for as long
as human history has been recorded. As we noted in the Preface,
for most of history, mankind managed to marginalize those who
were different from the mainstream of society. Many people with
IDD during most of the 19th Century and the first half of the 20th
Century were placed as children in large residential facilities when
their care at home proved difficult for their families (Scheerenberger, 1987). New York State was a leader in developing such residential facilities, which were called State Schools (Stearns, 2011).
Although initially well-run and well-funded, by the middle of the
20th Century, State Schools became overcrowded and under-
funded. Moreover, because of the lack of community alternatives,
placement in a State School guaranteed people would have almost
no chance to be reintegrated into society and lead productive
lives. Instead, they were vulnerable to poor health and early deaths
(Noll & Trent, 2004). No matter how well-run or well-funded the
State School System, the concept itself was degrading and abhor-
rent and its implementation inhumane in the lens of modern

history. One early, openly stated objective of the State School network was to reduce the incidence and prevalence of IDD in the general population by application of approaches such as eugenics (Pierson, 1893). Eugenics is the concept that controlled breeding can improve a human population to increase desirable traits. Developed largely by Francis Galton as a method of improving humanity, the concept of eugenics fell into disfavor only after the perversion of its doctrines by the Nazis.

Two residential institutions were in the Finger Lakes region through the late 19th and early 20th Centuries. In Newark, the New York State Custodial Asylum for Feeble-Minded Women opened in 1885.It was later renamed the Newark State School (State of New York Board of Charities Report, 1879). The Craig Colony for Epileptics (initially named the State of New York Epilepsy Asylum) opened in 1896 in the Town of Sonyea, an acronym derived from the first letters of each word in the institution's name. It was one of two facilities in the United States devoted to serving people with epilepsy (Stearns, 2011). By the time both facilities were closed, they housed over 5,000 people, many of whom did not originally reside in western New York.

Concern among families grew throughout the first half of the twentieth century about the lack of community-based services as well as discontent over the conditions in State Schools. In the 1940s and 1950s, parent groups formed all over the US and began to build a not-for-profit network of community-based services and supports for children and adults with IDD (Sheerenberger, 1987). Three organizations were formed in Rochester that would provide an alternative for parents who did not wish their children with IDD, who were receiving little or no education through public schools, to be admitted to a State School. The Association for Retarded Children (now the Arc of Monroe) was founded in 1958, the Day Care Center for Handicapped Children (now the Mary Cariola Children's Center) in 1949, and the Cerebral Palsy Association (now CP Rochester) in 1946. These three agencies began in different community locations but moved to the Al Sigl Center on Elmwood Avenue when it opened in 1968. The School of the Holy Childhood, a nonsectarian private school, also opened in Rochester in the mid-1940s. These and other private, not-for-profit agencies that opened their doors in the region offered only day programming; some provided children's educational services, and some offered adult programs. These agencies had in common the goal of responding to the substantial gaps in the continuum of community-based day-program options for children and adults with special needs. Collectively, they formed the bulwark needed to pursue full inclusion of people with IDD in mainstream society; this would not come until much later and is still evolving. Also, it was not until much later that group homes and other small residential services appeared. The Rochester community will always be considered among the most progressive locales in the US in the development of not-for-profit agencies.

In the 1960s, New York State embarked upon a major expansion of its State School network, by now renamed as Developmental Centers. This initiative was intended to reduce overcrowding in existing State Schools and respond to increasing numbers of children and young adults with IDD for whom there were no residential alternatives (Stearns, 2011). A new facility was constructed on Westfall Road in Rochester and named the Monroe Developmental Center. New York State then adopted a plan to repatriate residents of State Schools to the facility nearest to their original home. Hence, the new beds at the Monroe Developmental Center were in immediate demand. At the same time, legal proceedings began across the United States to improve care in residential facilities, including a case brought against New York State on behalf of residents of The Willowbrook State School on Staten Island. This case resulted in a Consent Decree mandating several changes that would result in the beginning of a movement to deinstitutionalize people living in State Schools. Community settings were not yet ready to serve as an alternative; but the seeds were sown that assured success soon.

# Chapter Two

# LAYING A FOUNDATION

*Community pediatrics [has sought] to provide a far more realistic
and complete clinical picture by taking responsibility for all children in a community, providing preventive and curative services,
and understanding the determinants and consequences of child
health and illness, as well as the effectiveness of services provided.
Thus, the unique feature of community pediatrics is its concern
for all of the population—those who remain well but need preventive services, those who have symptoms but do not receive effective
care, and those who do seek medical care either in a physician's
office or in a hospital.*

— Robert Haggerty, 1994

Efforts to address the growing needs of parents of children with
IDD started at the University of Rochester in the late 1940s by
providing diagnostic services and community outreach and consultation. At first, separate clinical and teaching programs were
responsive to consumer needs, regarding both developmental and
behavioral concerns. The Department of Pediatrics served as the
venue for both program strands. Both strands evolved in different directions and were encouraged and supported by William
Bradford, MD, second Chair of the Department. Both strands also
included partnerships between academic medicine, allied health
disciplines such as psychology, education physical therapy and
other community-based initiatives. Both strands were built upon
the foundation of Community Pediatrics, of which the University of Rochester is considered a pioneer. Community Pediatrics
embodied a shift in child health care away from hospital-based
practice to a model that placed the child and his or her family
residing in a community setting at the center of decision-making
(Haggerty, 1968).

## Developmental Pediatrics

Ambulatory developmental diagnostic services were established by Wilbur K. Smith, MD. Dr. Smith was a neuroanatomist in the Department of Anatomy. In 1947 Dr. Bradford recruited him to the Department of Pediatrics and asked him to develop clinical services in child neurology, well before child neurology emerged as a specialty in medical schools around the United States. Dr. Smith mentored two pediatric neurology trainees, Agneta Borgstedt, MD, and Sandra Feldman, MD, and the three physicians established the first developmental evaluation clinic for IDD at URMC. A wide range of neurodevelopmental disorders were represented among referrals to the clinic, including IDD. Dr. Borgstedt left URMC in 1971 and established a community-based pediatric neurology practice specializing in learning disabilities, Attention Deficit Disorders, and Attention-Deficit/Hyperactivity Disorders.

Dr. Smith's clinic grew because of contributions by three consecutive chief residents in Pediatrics: Dr. Albert P. Scheiner (1957–58), Dr. Neal A. McNabb (1958–59), and Dr. William G. Kenney (1959–60). After completing their residences and stints in the US Air Force, Drs. Scheiner and McNabb were founding partners of the Panorama Pediatrics practice in Penfield, New York. In early 1961, Dr. Bradford asked Drs. Scheiner and McNabb to establish

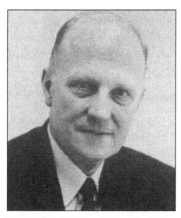

Figure 2.1. Wilber K. Smith, MD. Photo from Gary J. Myers, MD, and reproduced with permission.

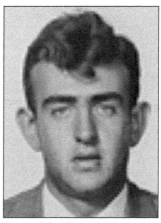

Figure 2.2. Albert P. Scheiner, MD.

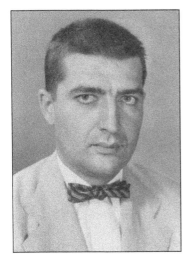

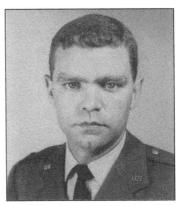

Figure 2.4. William G. Kenney, MD.

Figure 2.3. Neal A. McNabb, MD. Reproduced with permission.

a formal clinical program serving children and adolescents with IDD and learning disorders at the Strong Memorial Hospital Outpatient Clinic. In 1968, Drs. Scheiner and McNabb left private practice to devote full time to this venture. With New York State funding, they founded the Monroe Developmental Service as a community-based diagnostic and consultation clinic based at 797 Elmwood Avenue (*Children*, 1970, p. 240). They also obtained funding from Monroe County to establish the Diagnostic Clinic for Developmental Disorders (DCDD) at URMC.

The DCDD was headed by Dr. Kenney, Rune Simeonsson, PhD, was its psychologist, and Dorothy "Dotty" Jansma, EdM, provided educational evaluations.

The DCDD ran in tandem with two other clinics at URMC, both established in the late 1960s. These were the Learning Disabilities Clinic, an interdisciplinary diagnostic service run by D. Wilson "Bill" Hess, PhD, and Ellsworth "Babe" Westehoff, EdD, and the Birth Defects Center (BDC), an interdisciplinary service primarily focusing on the care of children with spina bifida and other neural tube defects. The BDC was initially funded by the March of Dimes and run by Paul Yudkofski, MD, and Gary J. Myers, MD, took over leadership of the BDC in the early 1970s, assisted by

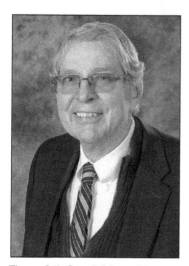

Figure 2.5. Gary J. Myers, MD. Photo from Dr. Myers and reproduced with permission.

Artis Olsen, MD. Following Dr. Myers' departure for the University of Alabama in 1978, he was succeeded first by Margaret Colgan, MD, and then by Gregory Liptak, MD, MPH (about whom we will have more to say later). The first BDC nurse was Sharon Bidwell Cerone, MSN, PhD, RN, who was succeeded by Gail Revell, MSN, RN.

In addition to serving the clinical needs of children and adolescents with spina bifida and their families, BDC faculty member Martha Gram, BS, RPT, collaborated with Edwin Kinnen, PhD, a member of the University of Rochester College of Engineering faculty, to develop devices that would enhance the function of children with spina bifida. This group built the Rochester Parapodium, a standing brace that allowed children with Spina Bifida or other spinal lesions causing paraplegia to navigate about their environment by movement of their torsos. The brace was designed to hold the child upright and had a flat bottom that provided stability and allowed the children to move through upper body rotation. It differed from earlier versions developed elsewhere in that it had knee and leg locks that permitted its user to sit and stand while wearing the device (Brown, Gram, & Kinnen, 1980). This was one of the earliest examples of biomedical engineering applied to children with physical disabilities. The Parapodium was patented but never produced commercially. Units were made by hand in Professor Kinnen's laboratory and distributed free of charge to children who would benefit from them.

Dr. Kinnen volunteered his time with the BDC. The program also benefited from volunteer services during the weekly clinics from several surgical subspecialists, without whose expertise, multidisciplinary care could not have been provided. These included neurosurgeons Joseph M. McDonald, MD, Shige-hisa Okawara, MD, and later Webster Pilcher, MD, PhD, and Paul Maurer, MD; Urologist Irwin Frank, MD, and later Ronald Rabinowitz, MD; Pedodontist Odd B. Sveen, DDS, PhD, and later Steven M. Adair, DDS, MS; orthotists Robert Nitschte and Gerald Tinsdale from the Rochester Orthopaedics Laboratory; and orthopedists Peter Haake, MD, William Bogart, MD, Franklin V. Peale, MD, and later Thomas Putnam, MD, and Kenneth "Van" Jackman, MD.

Before he left URMC, Dr. Myers collaborated with Drs. Cerone and Olsen to publish a guide for parents of children with spina bifida (Myers et al., 1981). This guide is still available. The BDC also engaged volunteers, some of whom had spina bifida, who attended BDC clinics and were available to parents of clinic services consumers for informal chats. They also oversaw a small mobile lending library cart with materials such as the Myers, Cerone, and Olsen guide.

## Behavioral Pediatrics

The impetus for developing clinical and teaching programs in behavioral pediatrics began when Dr. Bradford recruited Stanford B. Friedman, MD, a pediatrician and a graduate of the University of Rochester School of Medicine and Dentistry, who was interested in the interaction of behavior and biologic illness. Dr. Friedman trained under Dr. George Engel, who is widely regarded as the physician who recognized the bidirectional effect of psychosocial issues and health. Dr. Friedman was charged with establishing behavioral approaches within pediatric care at URMC (Sharkey, 2013). The behavioral pediatrics strand received a big boost from the recruitment in 1964 of Robert J. Haggerty, MD, as chair of Pediatrics to succeed Dr. Bradford (Haggerty & Aligne, 2005; Haggerty & Friedman, 2003). Dr. Haggerty was considered a leader in the promotion of Community Pediatrics (Haggerty, 1968; 1994). He was also considered a visionary in the promotion of behavioral interaction with health and recognition of such in the goals of Community Pediatrics as an academic entity. Drs.

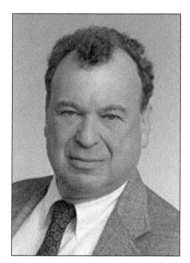

Figure 2.6. Stanford B. Friedman, MD. Reproduced with permission.

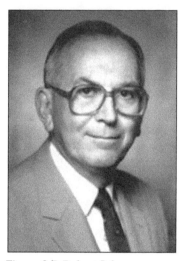

Figure 2.7. Robert Johns Haggerty, MD. Reproduced with permission.

Friedman and Haggerty are jointly credited with founding the field of behavioral pediatrics; however, the term *behavioral pediatrics* was first published in a now-famous editorial by Dr. Friedman in the *Journal of Pediatrics* (Friedman, 1970).

Behavioral consultations were established for inpatient and ambulatory services and a training program was created. The training program graduated seven fellows in behavioral pediatrics in its first 10 years, including Philip Nader, MD, Sam Yancy, MD, and Elizabeth R. McAnarney MD, all of whom went on to distinguished careers in Adolescent Medicine. Dr. Friedman also established an adolescent clinic that served as a venue for teaching and service, a school health program, and numerous research projects. Additional pediatric faculty members joined these efforts, including Barry Pless, MD, Robert Chamberlin, MD, Evan Charney, MD, James Heriot, PhD, Klaus Roghmann, PhD, James Perrin, MD, and Ellen Perrin, MD. Drs. Nader and McAnarney remained on the faculty following completion of their fellowships. Winifred Stebbens, EdM, was a Special Educator who provided both direct service and resident teaching around children with learning problems who were receiving their primary care at URMC. Salary support and fellowship stipends were funded by two grants from the Children's Bureau (now known as the Maternal and Child Health Bureau [MCHB]). These efforts collectively gave identity to behavioral pediatrics as a special focus within pediatrics and firmly established the concept that psychosocial factors played a substantial role in children's health and development.

# Chapter Three

# OPPORTUNITIES

*We can say with some assurance that, although children may be the victims of fate, they will not be the victims of our neglect.*

—John F. Kennedy, remarks upon signing the Maternal and Child Health and Mental Retardation Planning Bill, October 24, 1963

Federal support of university-based training regarding IDD dates back to the passage of the Social Security Act of 1935. That legislation contained the Maternal and Child Health Service Block Grant (also known as Title V of the Social Security Act), which created the Maternal and Child Health Bureau (MCHB). The goals of the MCHB were to support public health efforts to reduce infant mortality and the incidence of handicapping conditions; to provide and assure access to rehabilitation services to children with disabilities; and to help to develop comprehensive, family-centered, community-based, culturally competent, coordinated systems of services for children with special health care needs and their families. Federal support for services to children and adults with IDD grew during the 1940s and 1950s along with the Civil Rights movement (Scheerenberger, 1987).

During the administration of John F. Kennedy, the President's Panel on Mental Retardation [sic] was created as an advisory group to the President. The President's sister Rosemary had mild IDD until she was in her twenties, when she had a prefrontal lobotomy and was left severely disabled for the remainder of her life (Larson, 2015). Thus, President Kennedy was aware of the importance of developing and maintaining services and supports for people with IDD. This step marked the first time that IDD received attention from high levels of the US federal government.

In its initial reports to the President (President's Panel on Mental Retardation, 1963), the Panel recognized the need for federally funded programs to improve the quality of service delivery to people with IDD and to increase training opportunities available to professionals in the field of IDD services. The Mental Retardation Facilities and Community Health Centers Construction Act of 1963 (Public Law 88–164) was the first public law guaranteeing services to persons with developmental disabilities. It authorized the University Affiliated Facilities (UAF) Program to provide core and administrative funds to improve training opportunities as well as facilitate the development of service models to provide care to people with IDD. However, UAFs were not authorized to use core and administrative funds to support direct clinical services. The law mandated that UAFs created through its funding be colocated and affiliated with major institutions of higher learning, and that a commitment be made to the training of professional workers in an interdisciplinary program to be able to advocate and develop exemplary services for persons who had IDD. In addition, the plan called for the establishment of a number of these centers to create a nationwide network. Initially, 10 facilities were constructed with federal monies, administered by the Developmental Disabilities Office (DDO) in the US Department of Health and Human Services. An additional six universities received UAF grants but not construction funds. This network subsequently grew and now numbers 67 centers in the United States, at least one in every state and territory (Association of University Centers on Disabilities, https://www.aucd.org/docs/publications/brochures/ucedd_brochure2006_withinsert.pdf) but it would take many years for the network to grow and it would be some time before URMC amassed the resources to compete for these funds.

UAFs were expected to be a bridge between the university and the community. Member sites of the UAF network had the opportunity to apply for targeted grant funding to accomplish this mission. This included Leadership Education in Neurodevelopmental and Related Disorders (LEND) interdisciplinary training program funded by grants from MCHB. Not all UAFs were approved for funding as LEND programs. The US Department of Education made teacher preparation funds available to UAFs. Federal matching funds were also made available for construction of facilities to house programs funded under a facilities construction act, giving rise to the term University Affiliated Facility. By the early 1980s, the Administration on Developmental Disabilities (ADD; formerly the DDO) renamed the UAFs as University Affiliated Programs (UAPs), recognizing that the recent and anticipated expansion of the federal mandate would no longer include construction funds. Later, the nomenclature was again changed to University Centers of Excellence in Developmental Disabilities (UCEDDs).

President Kennedy's administration was advised by Robert Cooke, MD, chairperson of Pediatrics at the Johns Hopkins University at that time, who himself was the father of two offspring with profound IDD (Robert E. Cooke Obituary, The Johns Hopkins Medical Institutions, 2014; The Alan Mason Chesney Medical Archives of The Johns Hopkins Medical Institutions, https://medicalarchives.jhmi.edu:8443/papers/cooke.html). Dr. Cooke knew that research into the causes of and innovative treatments for children (and adults) with IDD was lacking. He urged President Kennedy to propose a special program to be funded by the National Institute of Child Health and Human Development (NICHD) that created Mental Retardation and Developmental Disabilities Research Centers (MRDDRCs, now named Intellectual and Developmental Disabilities Research Centers or IDDRCs). These grants provided core and administrative support to programs already engaged in research on IDD. All the initial 16 recipient institutions of higher learning of MRDDRC grants were holders of UCEDD grants, even though the authorizing legislation made no mention of such colocation. This program has been maintained by NICHD but limited to 16 centers that now compete for renewal funding every five years assuring some turnover in the sites funded.

# Chapter Four

# CHANGING OF THE GUARD

*Change will not come if we wait for some other person, or if we wait for some other time. We are the ones we've been waiting for. We are the change that we seek.*

—Barack Obama

A change occurred in the University of Rochester faculty by 1974. Dr. Haggerty moved first to Harvard, and then assumed the presidency of the W. T. Grant Foundation. Dr. Friedman moved to the University of Maryland's College of Medicine. Drs. Scheiner and McNabb remained in Rochester but left private practice to expand the Monroe Developmental Service into the Monroe Developmental Center (MDC). Their vision was to use the newly constructed building on Westfall Road as a resource for day-habilitation services rather than fill the over-500 beds the building was designed to accommodate. The New York State Office of Mental Retardation and Developmental Disabilities or OMRDD (known now as The Office for People with Developmental Disabilities, or OPWDD) disagreed and exerted great pressure on MDC leadership and eventually prevailed. MDC's first resident was an adult who moved from Newark State School and was admitted in 1975. Dr. Scheiner worked to obtain federal funding to support a community-university collaborative center addressing service, education, and research on IDD; but this vision did not gain momentum locally and funding was not sought to establish a comprehensive center for IDD at the University of Rochester at that time. Dr. Scheiner's commitment to following the principles of Normalization (Wolfensberger et al., 1972) fit very well with the Community Pediatrics model and formed the basis for what was to come next.

In 1976, Dr. Scheiner moved to the University of Massachusetts Medical School in Worcester at the invitation of J. Barry

Hanshaw, MD, a Rochester colleague who had become chairperson of Pediatrics there. Dr. McNabb stayed on at MDC and provided leadership as the new residential facility on Westfall Road opened its doors and accepted many people who had been placed in communal care facilities in other parts of New York State. Dr. McNabb left MDC in 1978 but remained in Rochester to head the Pediatric Service at the Genesee Hospital and establish the Genesee Developmental Unit. This clinical entity provided diagnostic evaluations to children and adolescents with suspected IDD. Dr. Kenney also moved to MDC but remained active at the DCDD as well. Drs. Chamberlin, Nader, Charney, and Heriot also left Rochester; Dr. Roghmann remained.

Some important new additions to the Department of Pediatrics occurred during this period that would have an impact on the increasing focus on behavioral and developmental pediatrics in the Department of Pediatrics. Stanley Novak, MD, replaced Dr. Nader as director of the School Health Programs, Christopher Hodgman, MD, a child and adolescent psychiatrist, assumed some of the clinical roles filled by Dr. Friedman, including an expansion of the Consultation-Liaison Service. Dr. McAnarney was named director of the Division of Adolescent Medicine, thus assuring an academic base for biopsychosocial medicine for adolescents. She was joined by Ollie Jane Sahler, MD, who as a medical student had worked with Dr. Friedman. Dr. Sahler completed an Adolescent Medicine Fellowship with Drs. Hodgman and McAnarney.

With the departure of Dr. Haggerty as chair, David H. Smith, MD, a specialist in pediatric infectious disease, was recruited from Harvard Medical School to become the fourth chair of the Department in 1976 (URMC website, https://www.urmc.rochester.edu/cvbi/history.aspx). Philip W. Davidson, PhD, a pediatric psychologist with specialization in IDD arrived in 1974 to work at MDC with a part-time appointment in Pediatrics as a consultant to the School Health Programs. He moved full time to the DCDD in 1976, replacing Dr. Simeonsson, who moved to the University of North Carolina at Chapel Hill (UNC-CH). The nearly coincidental arrival of Drs. Smith and Davidson in 1976 would serendipitously accelerate the organization of a focus on IDD within not only Pediatrics, but also in other units of the University of Rochester. Dr. Smith had attended medical school at the University of Rochester and had early exposure to community pediatrics while studying with Dr. Engel. He understood the importance of psychosocial influences on child health and soon after his arrival in Rochester he began a departmental review that included behavioral and developmental pediatrics. He invited T. Berry Brazelton, MD, a noted expert in child development and behavior, to serve as an outside consultant in this review. It was clear from Dr. Brazelton's visit that he saw potential for some expansion of these subspecialties.

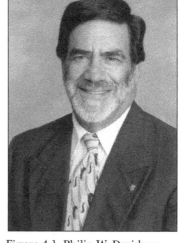

Figure 4.1. Philip W. Davidson, PhD.

Dr. Davidson had trained with Harrie Chamberlain, MD, Donald K. Routh, PhD, Carolyn S. Schroeder, PhD, and Stephen R. Schroeder, PhD, as a LEND Fellow at the Division for Disorders in Development and Learning (DDDL), a UCEDD at the UNC-CH, which also was funded for an IDDRC. He believed that a program could be built in Rochester that had all of the components he had seen in Chapel Hill; but he was also aware that one of the most direct ways to start was to seek funding, specifically for a UCEDD. It would be many years before URMC would be able to compete for either a LEND training grant or an IDDRC.

# Chapter Five

# EMERGENCE OF FOCUS

*Concentrate all your thoughts upon the work at hand.*
*The sun's rays do not burn until brought to a focus.*
—Alexander Graham Bell

The original group of UCEDDs was limited in number and no new UCEDDs were added through the 1970s. In 1977 DDO issued a call for proposals for feasibility studies to create five new UCEDDs, each of which would be tied to an existing UCEDD. They would be called UAF Satellite Centers. Dr. Davidson approached Allen C. Crocker, MD, director of the Developmental Evaluation Clinic, the UCEDD at Boston Children's Hospital, to discuss an application for a UAF Satellite Center in Rochester. Drs. Smith and Crocker knew each other well and had been research collaborators at Harvard. With Dr. Smith's encouragement, Drs. Crocker and Davidson applied for a UAF Satellite Feasibility Study that was funded in 1977. The Feasibility Study included a regionwide needs assessment that built the foundation for a strong link between the Medical Center and the Community. It also enabled collaborations between the Department of Pediatrics, otherMedical Centers, other units of the University of Rochester, or other local university departments to create an interdisciplinary team. In 1978, DDO funded Rochester and four other applicants as Satellite Centers, including programs in Vermont, Montana, Hawaii, and the Navaho Nation. All these programs had the missions of developing training and exemplary services in IDD for their regions, to provide technical assistance to their communities and to disseminate evidence-based information pertaining to best practices. (In later iterations of federal mandates, the requirement for dissemination was expanded to include applied research designed to improve the delivery of services and supports). No new Feasibility Study grants

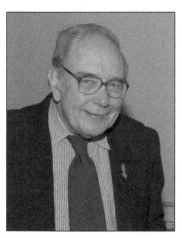

Figure 5.1. Allen C. Crocker, MD.

were made until 1984 (Davidson & Fifield, 1985); so, Rochester's timing was fortuitous.

The DCDD was renamed the University Affiliated DCDD or UADCDD in 1978. Dr. Davidson was the Principal Investigator and the primary psychologist. The original group was comprised of a combination of DCDD faculty members William G. Kenney. MD (Pediatrics), and Ms. Jansma (Education), with School Health Programs personnel Ruth J. Rockowitz (now Messinger), ACSW (Social Work), and Christine M. Burns, EdM, MBA (Education). Bretna Griffith, BS, was designated Regional Resources Coordinator for community technical assistance and outreach training; Marilyn "Lyn" Wiles-Kettenmann, MA, Research Coordinator; and Kathleen "Kathy" Wright (now Sweetland), Consumer Care Coordinator. Barbara Stern, MA (Speech Pathology); Sharon Bidwell Cerone, PhD, MSN, RN; Joy Quintero, OTR; Jorge Davila, DDS (Dentistry); and Reverend William Gaventa (Chaplaincy) also joined the team (Dr. Davidson, Rev. Gaventa, and Ms. Stern had all been colleagues at UNC-CH).

In 1981, the Rochester Program, which had remained a satellite of the Boston Children's Hospital UCEDD, became a full member of the American Association of University Affiliated Programs for Persons with Developmental Disabilities, now known as the Association of University Centers on Disabilities or AUCD. The AUCD is the professional organization of UCEDDs, IDDRCs, and other university-based disability programs. Membership meant recognition as a partner, but it also provided a window to information that could lead to growth of individual member centers. Election to full membership gave the Rochester UCEDD a voice in the development of the national IDD program and also afforded it with technical assistance toward its own development.

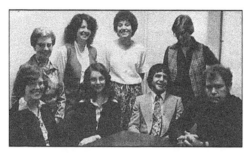

Figure 5.2. Several original UAP Satellite Center faculty and staff members (1978). Front row (*from left*) Pauline Young (secretary), Dorothy "Dottie" Jansma, EdM, (Special Education), Dr. Davidson, Dr. Kenney. Back row: Ona Lyman (secretary), Marilyn "Lyn" Wiles-Kettenmann, MA (research coordinator), Katherine "Kathy" Wright (patient coordinator), and Bretna Griffith (regional resources coordinator). Reproduced with permission from *Child Health*, Spring, 1978.

In 1981 the UCEDD was also designated an official division in the Department of Pediatrics with Dr. Davidson as Division Chief. This extended the original clinical service addressing developmental pediatric needs for evaluation to the training and community outreach requirements of the federal UCEDD network. The program was renamed as the University Affiliated Program in Developmental Disabilities or UAPDD. In 1988, ADD designated the University of Rochester program as a full UCEDD. The name was changed once again in 1992, to the Strong Center for Developmental Disabilities (SCDD).

Elevation to full UCEDD status brought parity with other UCEDD programs, and also meant a sizeable increase in annual federal funding. The interactions with other UCEDDs enabled sharing of ideas and allowed problem-solving to enhance growth in Rochester. The additional funds permitted the addition of more compensated time and effort from a larger number of faculty members and assisted the new UCEDD in approaching a critical mass. It enabled the development of affiliations with academic departments within the University of Rochester. It also facilitated formation of affiliations with academic departments outside the University of Rochester, which were necessary in cases where disciplines lacked a local academic home.

When SCDD was designated a full UCEDD, the formal relationship between Rochester and Boston ended. Dr. Crocker remained a good friend to Rochester and to the SCDD until his passing in 2011. His contributions to developmental and behavioral pediatrics and, more broadly, to IDD in Western New York, were then and remain now immeasurable.

# Chapter Six

# TEAM BUILDING

*Alone we can do so little, together we can do so much.*
—Helen Keller

The Rochester UCEDD's initial team was composed of some faculty members who were committed to devoting significant time to the new program, but others were not, and new leadership was required. Recruitment of faculty from other UCEDDs was a high priority. But recruitment of partners from community agencies also took place. SCDD concentrated on establishing a governance structure, and on building an exemplary service and support base upon which a training program could be built, and ultimately upon which outcome research could be conducted.

The governance structure was traditional for UCEDDs. Dr. Davidson appointed directors of exemplary service, preservice training, community outreach, and dissemination. This group formed an Executive Committee to oversee program development. This leadership team structure persists to this day, with the updating of functional groupings to Clinical Services, Training, Community Programs, Research, and Administration and Finance.

## Leadership Recruitment

No individuals were more important to these efforts than Christine M. Burns, EdM, MBA, and Ruth J. Messinger, ACSW. Dr. Davidson had worked with both on the School Health Programs team and they shared the same values and visions. When the UCEDD Satellite Center was funded, Dr. Davidson turned to both for help in shaping the new program. Both understood interdisciplinary training and had been involved in various ways with pediatric resident education prior to Dr. Davidson's arrival in Rochester. Both knew the disability community and how to bring the new UCEDD closer to community-based programs. Both were excellent clinicians and were committed to improving services for children with IDD and complex health care needs. However, they had different foci and different skill sets.

Ruth Messinger made a major contribution to the field by developing programs supporting individuals with IDD who became involved with the criminal justice system. In the late 1970s and early 1980s, the deinstitutionalization movement increased the number of people with IDD living in the community but did not provide the necessary supports and services to deal with behavioral problems. In some cases, this led to interactions with the criminal justice system, which was not prepared for addressing such consumers' needs. Cultural differences between the service systems needed to be addressed and few locales were ready to do so. Ms. Messinger conceived an approach that utilized a community task force to define a program to divert adults with IDD from incarceration. This led to the development of the Rochester Alleged Offender Program, which became a national model for best practice (see Chapter 7). Later in her career, Ms. Messinger served as LEND Social Work Coordinator for the UCEDD, chair of the Strong Memorial Hospital Child Protection Committee and chief social worker in Pediatrics. She assisted with the development and implementation of the newly awarded (1997) MCHB-funded Interdisciplinary Training in Adolescent Health Program grant directed by Richard Kriepe, MD, at URMC.

Christine Burns's career spanned 42 years. It was focused on three related but distinct spheres: coordination of care for children with special health care needs and their families, health-care provider education and training, and health-care financing and management.

Ms. Burns was the Associate Director for Finance and Administration and, later, the Associate Chief of the Division. She was an expert on finance, long-range planning, and administration. In 1996, she joined the Department of Pediatrics central administration half-time, and pursued both finance and administration; she used her passion to create a coordination-of-care program. Working with Department of Pediatrics Administrator Elizabeth

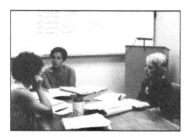

Figure 6.1. Ruth J. Messinger, ACSW (*right*), with Christine M. Burns, EdM, MBA (*center*) and a trainee. Photo from SCDD archives and reproduced with permission.

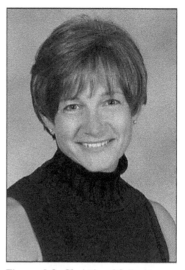

Figure 6.2. Christine M. Burns, EdM, MBA. Photo from Thomas R. Burns Esq and reproduced with permission.

Lattimore, Ms. Burns helped to redesign pediatric ambulatory care.

In 1978, Francis "Frank" Bennett, PhD, was recruited from the Nisonger Center UCEDD at the Ohio State University to head the Psychology discipline. He and Dr. Davidson worked together to develop predoctoral and postdoctoral training programs in Pediatric Psychology; trainees and fellows were recruited soon thereafter. Some early fellows, such as Bonnie Kwiatkowski Kramer, PhD, and Lori Jean Peloquin, PhD, remained on the faculty after completing their fellowship training and then continued to practice in the Rochester area. Dr. Bennet left the UCEDD after only five years to pursue a private practice in Rochester, where he still resides. Following his departure, several UCEDD faculty members served as discipline coordinators for psychology and continued the training of postdoctoral fellows. These include Christine Chandler, PhD, Lori Jean Peloquin, PhD, and Karin Theurer-Kaufman, PhD. The fellowship continues today under the leadership of Laura Silverman, PhD.

In 1979, Ronald W. Schworm, PhD, was recruited from the State University of New York at Albany to join the UCEDD. Dr. Schworm was a special educator with a research interest in reading disorders and held a joint appointment in the Margaret Warner

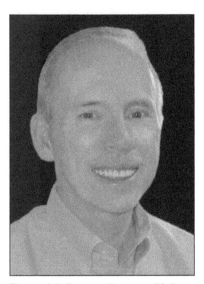

Figure 6.3. Frances Bennett, Ph.D. Photo from Dr. Bennett and reproduced with permission.

Graduate School of Education and Human Development and the Department of Pediatrics. Almost immediately, Dr. Schworm began work on a training grant application for teacher preparation, which was awarded in 1980 for three years of funding by the Office of Special Education Resources and Services (OSERS), US Department of Education. This grant paved the way for interdisciplinary training of special education graduate students in the new UAF Satellite Center. Dr. Schworm left the University of Rochester in 1986 for private practice in Rochester following the end of the second three-year funding cycle for his training grant. Although with the SCDD for only a short period, Dr. Schworm's tireless efforts to build a partnership between URMC and the Warner Graduate School of Education and Human Development laid the foundation for future collaborative projects, which continue today.

Stephen B. Sulkes, MD, joined the URMC faculty in 1984. Dr. Sulkes arrived in Rochester in 1983 following completion of his fellowship training with Dr. Allen Crocker at Boston Children's Hospital. He first accepted a position at the Monroe Developmental Center. He moved to SCDD after one year, but not before developing a very good network of ties to local agencies, including the Arc of Monroe County. By 1986, Dr. Sulkes had arranged for a half-time position for himself between the Arc of Monroe and SCDD. Dr. Sulkes was the first fellowship-trained Developmental Pediatrician in SCDD's history. He went on to serve as SCDD Discipline Coordinator for Pediatrics and directed divisional training programs (described further on). In 2006, he succeeded Dr.

Davidson as UCEDD director. Dr. Sulkes served as Director of Training for the Division of Developmental and Behavioral Pediatrics through 2019, and led the rotation in DBP required of all pediatric and medicine-pediatrics residents until 2019, when he passed leadership to Abigail Kroening, MD. He is the director of the American College of Graduate Medical Education (ACGME) Fellowship program in Developmental Behavioral Pediatrics. He worked closely with the Healthy Athletes Program of Special Olympics and was honored for his efforts at the

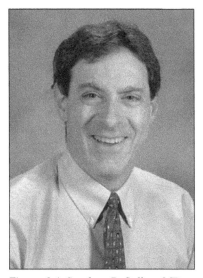

Figure 6.4. Stephen B. Sulkes, MD. Photo from SCDD archives and reproduced with permission.

international meeting in 2018. Dr. Sulkes' funded research collaborations included a Centers for Disease Control and Prevention special initiative to determine if there was an increased risk for Autism Spectrum Disorders (ASD) in youth with Down syndrome and projects related to health care utilization by people with IDD.

Dr. Schworm was succeeded as discipline coordinator for Education by Susan Hetherington, PhD, one of his first students. Dr. Hetherington, a former first-grade and resource-room teacher, participated in Dr. Schworm's OSERS-funded EdM program and after receiving her degree, she continued to teach at the Warner School while joining the UCEDD faculty. She held joint faculty appointments in Pediatrics and Education since 1983 and played a key role as a bridge between SCDD and the Warner School. Dr. Hetherington has more than 40 years' experience working with people with IDD, administering state and national grants, and training teachers and related services personnel. Her research interests include the social construction of disability and disability categories, the development of inclusive schools, transition to adulthood and employment of adults with IDD, and the intersection of race and disability. She wrote and received funding for a variety of grants from OSERS, the Administration for Intellectual and Developmental Disabilities (AIDD—the successor to the DDO), the NYS Department of Health, and the NYS OPWDD. Among these projects was an OSERS grant that provided funding for a facilitator-specialist training program to impact on the need for personnel to provide early intervention services. Patricia "Patti" Caro, EdS, served as project coordinator. This program established SCDD as a resource for early intervention training, serving as a companion to model service programs that were developing at SCDD at the time, and foreshadowing divisional research on early intervention, which we discuss further on.

Dr. Hetherington served as a member of the OPWDD Commissioner's Advisory Council and the NYS Rehabilitation Association Advisory Council. Dr. Hetherington also succeeded Dr. Davidson in representing the Rochester UCEDD as a member of the New York State Developmental Disabilities Planning Council (NYSDDPC). She consulted with several school districts around systemic issues related to inclusive classrooms and schools. Grant support has also included a NYS-funded project to support parent involvement in Early Intervention, a NYS grant to promote adult employment of people with IDD, and a collaborative study related to supports for health literacy of adolescents with ASD. Dr. Hetherington served as the UCEDD director for the last few years prior to her retirement in 2020. Among the many awards she received was the prestigious Dr. David Satcher Community Health Improvement Award for 2020.

## Advisory Boards

In 1985, SCDD created an Academic Advisory Board (AAB) and a Community Advisory Board (CAB). The AAB membership was composed of Department Chairs representing the various disciplines on SCDD's interdisciplinary faculty.

The CAB membership comprised key SCDD community constituencies, including self-advocates and their parents or other relatives, state and local voluntary agencies' directors, the New York

State Developmental Disabilities Planning Council and the New York State Protection and Advocacy System. The SCDD CAB predated Consumer Advisory Boards mandated for all UCEDDs by the federal Developmental Disabilities Bill of Rights and Assistance Act. Under requirement, SCDD changed the name of the CAB to the Consumer Advisory Council (CAC). The composition of the CAC was altered to accommodate a federal mandate of 50% consumers or consumer advocates. The CAC's first chair was Georgia McCabe. She

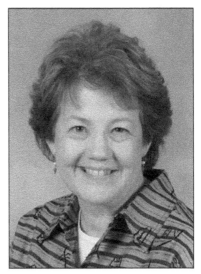

Figure 6.5. Susan Hetherington, PhD, reproduced with permission.

was succeeded by Teena Fitzroy, who also became a voting member of the SCDD Executive Committee. Ms. Fitzroy was succeeded by Joanne Armstrong, who chaired the CAC until she retired in 2010. It is now cochaired by Ann Scherff and Lindsay Jewett. The CAC has a significant impact on SCDD strategic planning and provides a crucial link to the IDD community. It continues to be an integral part of the SCDD governance structure.

## Contributions by Staff

The clinical, community, and training activities of the SCDD would not have been possible without dedicated staff who were enthusiastic about the shared mission. Between the 1970s and the present, administrative staff accounted for over a third of the Division's workforce. Over 100 people held administrative positions over the history of the Division. Some long-term team members from the formative years and through the years Dr. Davidson was division chief include: Bretna Griffith, Katherine Sweetland, Katherine

Purcell (who was later appointed to the faculty and served as manager of clinical operations), Marilyn Wiles-Kettenmann, Ona Lyman, Nancy Davidow, Joyce Goodberlet, Ginger Potter, Jean Reeves, Beatrice Fornieri, Elizabeth Schnucker, Lorraine McMullen, Gregory Coccitti, Bernadette Jackson, Carolyn King, Kathryn Cook, Phyllis Ives, Janet Ouimette and Catherine Imhof. Their contributions extended across service, training, and research programs, and included the administrative management of the Division.

Since Christine Burns stepped down from her position and Dr. Davidson retired as Division Chief, there have been three Directors of Finance and Administration. Michelle Casey, MPA, led the division through a comprehensive strategic planning process involving all faculty and staff that informed an overhaul of divisional internal policies and procedures with input from a wide representation of division members. Research activities were sufficient to create a position within the division for a research administrator. Norma Harary, PhD, held this position until her death in 2013. Marilee Montanaro, MBA, EdD, was the next Director of Administration and Finance. She led the division through the implementation of the strategic plan and helped streamline staffing through a redesigned management structure for efficiency across the division. She introduced modern accounting systems and improved divisional communication through use of technological advances. The second divisional research administrator, Berlin Bermudez, MMS, PhD, was succeeded by Melody Newman, MMS, during her administration. Peter (Mack) Kennedy, MBA, joined the division in July 2018 following the departure of Dr. Montanero. He had prior experience in administrative positions in research and behavioral health at the Cleveland Clinic and Cincinnati Children's Hospital and further integrated service lines and improved process and efficiency.

# Chapter Seven

# MATURATION

*Normalization is the utilization of means which are as cultur-*
*ally normative as possible, in order to establish and/or maintain*
*personal behaviors and characteristics which are as culturally*
*normative as possible.*
—Wolfensberger et al., 1972, p. 28

The changing ideology in the field of IDD significantly impacted the maturation of the Rochester UCEDD. At the heart of this ideological shift was the principle of Normalization. It was first defined in Sweden by Bengt Nirje (1969) and championed extensively in the United States and Canada by Wolf Wolfensberger (Wolfensberger et al., 1972). This principle was based upon the concept that people with IDD, no matter what their disability, would benefit by immersion into the most typical level of lifestyle they could manage. This philosophy formed the basis for the deinstitutionalization movement, followed by elimination of barriers to full inclusion in society. It would take decades and promulgation of some very important changes in federal civil rights legislation before old approaches to services and supports would give way to real change.

SCDD was not a self-contained unit with large resources when it became a UCEDD Satellite Center. Therefore, the ensuing program had to emerge through the judicious use of core resources to recruit collaborations and partnerships with colleagues and investigators from the University of Rochester, and from other higher education centers. Partnerships were also expanded with local and state providers and consumer groups, all of which had begun to move towards a focus on deinstitutionalization and normalization. These liaisons helped to extend the network and to develop funding bases, largely from state resources at first. By creatively sharing faculty and staff positions and governance with other agencies, permanent and systemic structures were eventually achieved.

## Postgraduate Training Programs

Clinical training in Developmental and Behavioral Pediatrics of medical students, residents, and fellows, mainly in the Departments of Pediatrics and Psychiatry, was underway during the 1960s and early 1970s. The receipt of federal UCEDD funds, however, enabled trainee and faculty support for interdisciplinary training, which quickly grew to include as many as 10 disciplines. As soon as the UCEDD Satellite Center was funded in 1978, Ms. Burns became the training director and a curriculum was developed composed of clinical rotations and a year-long credit-bearing core course. The first trainees included the disciplines of Psychology, Pediatrics, Social Work, Speech Language Pathology, and Nursing. All trainees were postgraduate students or postdoctoral fellows in the case of Psychology and Developmental Pediatrics.

Until Dr. Sulkes joined SCDD, medical education was undertaken by a cadre of part-time pediatricians who were also providing medical services in SCDD clinics, including Drs. Kenney, Thomas McInerny, Bruce Kleene, and Barton Kaplan. They were joined by Elmar Frangenberg, MD, who had trained in child neurology with Frederick Horner, MD, chief of the division of child neurology. Dr. Frangenberg served in medical director roles at the Monroe Developmental Center and CP Rochester while continuing at SCDD on a part-time basis.

With the arrival of Dr. Sulkes, SCDD was able to develop subspecialty fellowship training for pediatricians. As the State of New York began closing its Developmental Centers it recognized a need to train physicians in the community to care for individuals with IDD. In 1985 a plan was developed by NYS OPWDD in collaboration with the academic medical centers in New York State. The Consortium for Medical Education in Developmental Disabilities (C-MEDD) funded faculty and fellows. SCDD received one of these grants and created a program that included training pediatricians, dentists, and psychiatrists. The program was directed by Dr. Sulkes and continued until 1990. The model of split positions between

SCDD and community or state agencies was employed extensively over the next 20 years to fund trainees and faculty. This approach also permitted training to address lifespan issues from childhood to adulthood (Davidson et al., 1986).

Without comprehensive core and administrative costs coverage for trainee stipends and faculty salaries, SCDD's training program grew slowly. Between 1985 and 1997, a total of 586 trainees from between eight and 15 disciplines or majors received graduate or postgraduate training. Around 80 percent of trainees spent less than 300 hours per year in various SCDD training activities. Most trainees represented the disciplines of medicine, psychology, and education (see also Table 8.1).

## Exemplary Services and Supports

Ever since the 1950s SCDD's primary focus had been direct clinical services. When it became a UCEDD, this focus had to broaden to include demonstration of model services that could address unique needs in upstate New York and beyond. This meant seeking grant funds, establishing new programs, finding appropriate space, establishing program evaluation, providing in-service education, and undertaking dissemination of findings. Between 1978 and 1985, SCDD acquired funding to initiate some model interdisciplinary community-based services and supports. There were two distinct but intertwined themes underpinning these model programs: developing or enhancing capacity in rural areas, and coordination of services and supports. The goal was to provide evidence-based best practices. These programs included areas in both developmental and behavioral pediatrics and most were focused on young children and their families; but adult services began to emerge as an important new direction for SCDD.

A feature of many of the model programs developed during this period was the close collaboration between SCDD, other URMC units, and NYS OPWDD. Many programs were funded by grants from NYS OPWDD, some projects shared faculty and staff, and even shared governance. In a similar manner, some programs began with funding from the NYSDDPC and from the New York State Education Department (NYSED) and the New York State

Department of Health. Without this support and innovative service designs that resulted from it, SCDD would not have grown to the extent it did, nor would it have become as integrated into the disability community as it did.

## *Diagnostic Clinic for Developmental Disorders*

In 1985, SCDD absorbed the clinical services originally provided by the Learning Disorders Clinic. SCDD also undertook administrative management of the Birth Defects Center (BDC). Multidisciplinary evaluations took place for some children over multiple days, culminating in extensive interdisciplinary team discussions that included representatives from schools, community agencies, and parents. More streamlined bidisciplinary models (pediatrics and education) were developed for evaluation for possible ADHD. Despite the training value and clinical insights gained from large interdisciplinary models, these became unwieldy in the face of increasing demand and limited reimbursement, and more streamlined models were developed.

The need for ongoing management of behavioral challenges in children with IDD and limited access to psychiatrists in the community who had experience with IDD led to increasing clinical volumes of DCDD consumers requiring medication management. The evolution of nurse practitioners initially as physician extender and subsequently as independent clinical providers helped improve access for ongoing management of the complex medical needs of children and youth with IDD.

To promote the continuum of developmental care in the DCDD, the clinical entity was renamed first the Center for Developmental Assessment (CDA) and later became the Andrew J. Kirch Developmental Services Center. (We will have more to say about Mr. Kirch further on.) Clinic directors have included Ms. Burns and Dr. Hetherington. In 2006, Lynn Cole, MSN, PNP, became the Director of Clinical Services.

A grant from the NYSDDPC established a joint program of SCDD and the Division of Child Neurology, the Finger Lakes Convulsive Disorders Center (FLCDC). This was led by Frederick Horner, MD, for the three years of funding. Joan Chodosh, ACSW served as the project social worker. Upon his retirement, SCDD assumed administration of the division of child neurology with supervision by Margaret McBride, MD, until Leon Epstein, MD, was recruited in 1988 to be the division chief of child neurology. The project also linked with an inpatient seizure unit directed by Giuseppe Erba, MD, and eventually became a component of Dr. Erba's Comprehensive Epilepsy Program in the Department of Neurology.

### The Mobile Diagnostic Unit (MDU)

Dating to the early 1970s, SCDD provided outreach diagnostic services and consultations in the community. For example, weekly all-day visits (including developmental pediatrics, psychology, and special education) took place on-site at the School of the Holy Childhood. When the UCEDD Satellite Center was awarded, those funds were allocated for a Mobile Diagnostic Unit modeled after a consultation service developed by Dr. Kenney for the School of the Holy Childhood. Contracts were arranged with several community agencies in the Finger Lakes Region to which a group of six or seven faculty and their students traveled several times a year. Evaluations took place on-site in the community setting. In addition to the evaluations, feedback sessions were held with agency staff and families. Noontime educational offerings were provided. This service was very popular amongst faculty, students, parents, and providers; it continued until the early 1990s and formed a basis for the present-day Community Consultation Program.

### The Regional Early Childhood Direction Center (RECDC) and Neonatal Continuing Care Program (NCCP)

This project was developed jointly between SCDD and the Division of Neonatology, led by Donald Shapiro, MD. (Davidson et al., 1984). Financed by a contract with the Board of Cooperative Educational Services (BOCES) in Fairport, New York, from funds from the NYSED, its mission was to identify the needs of infants and toddlers age birth to five years with special educational needs stemming from a disability, and to match those needs to available services. Before the extension of services down to infancy under the revisions to the federal special education law (Individuals

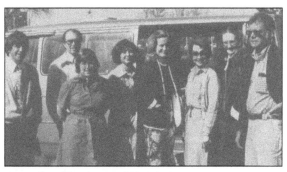

Figure 7.1. The Original Mobile Unit Team (*from left*):
Dr. Davidson, Dr. Schworm, Trainee Fitzgerald, Trainee
Carmola, Ms. Kennedy, Ms. Messinger, Drs. Bidwell-
Cerone and Kenney. Reproduced with permission
from *Child Health*, Fall, 1980.

with Disabilities Education Act, or IDEA) in 1992, early intervention and preschool service funding required filing of a Family
Court petition for each child. This was an important service pro-
vided by the RECDC, located in Fairport, New York, in a shopping
center 13 miles from Rochester. It was directed and coordinated
by Michael E. Reif, a BOCES employee who also served on the
SCDD faculty. Other founding staff included Mary Pinkerton, EdM
(Special Education), and Elizabeth Schnucker, MS (Social Work).
Ms. Pinkerton was later succeeded by Beatrice Fornieri, MS. The
RECDC also offered the Neonatal Continuing Care Program
(NCCP) based at URMC, which included a weekly clinic and a
tracking program to monitor developmental trends in infants and
children who had received neonatal intensive care services. Laurie Walsh RN, BSN, coordinated the NCCP. Dr. Davidson served
as the psychologist and Dr. Myers served as the child neurologist.
Margaret "Peggy" Oakes was the first Social Worker. Faculty members of the Division of Neonatology and Neonatology Fellows also
attended. The emergence of Early Intervention services under
Part H of the IDEA took place in the early 1990s, and many of
the coordination services of RECDC are now provided by Early
Intervention Programs of county Departments of Health. The current Infant and Toddler Program formed in 2012 succeeded the
NCCP as a joint clinical and training setting shared by SCDD and

the Division of Neonatology. It was directed by Robin Adair, MD, a Developmental Behavioral pediatrician with expertise in neonatal follow-up and infant behavioral health recruited from the University of Massachusetts until 2019. Medical leadership transitioned to Jessica Reiffer, MD, who received her fellowship training in Rochester. Psychology evaluations of high-risk infants transitioned from Dr. Davidson to Kelley Yost, PhD. Dr. Yost continued as co-PI of the NIH funded Neonatal Network Grant with Carl

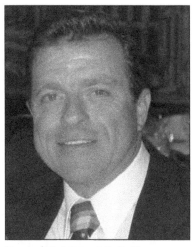

Figure 7.2. Michael E. Reif, MA. Photo from Mr. Reif and reproduced with permission.

D'Angio. MD, of the Division of Neonatology at URMC until 2020. He prepared Brenna Cavanaugh, Psy.D., to succeed him.

Michael Reif made substantial contributions to SDDD and to the disability community in general throughout his long career at BOCES. In 1986, Governor Mario Cuomo appointed him as Chairperson of the NYSDDPC, a position he held for five years. In 1985, he received a Jefferson Award for public service to the community from the City of Rochester.

## The Crisis Intervention Program (CI)

This project was developed jointly between SCDD and NYS OPWDD (Davidson et al., 1995). The initial study was supported by a grant for Category I Family Support Services and resulted from a Needs and Resources assessment that revealed several gaps in service for individuals with IDD who had recently been deinstitutionalized, or who were living with family members. The study was led by the late Leonard Salzman, PhD, of the Department of Psychiatry, Lori Jeanne Peloquin, PhD, and Dr. Davidson. The gaps that were identified included coordination of behavioral and mental health and disabilities services, emergency placement options, and staff training for management of behavior disorders, nonemergency respite options, and other crises.

Based upon this study, the NYS OPWDD organized a crisis service that was shared between the OPWDD's Finger Lakes Developmental Disabilities Services Office (FLDDSO) and the SCDD. Key to the implementation of this unique concept were the DDSO director, Sylvester P. Zielinski, and the DDSO director of community services, Marie O'Horo. The first director of the program was Trudy Fletcher, MSW, an administrator employed by the FLDDSO. She was succeeded by Virginia Giesow, MS, also an FLDDSO administrator who had done her fellowship in Speech Language Pathology at SCDD. The CI Program started serving consumers in April 1986 and was a model for implementation in other regions of NYS. The CI team reached its full capacity later in 1986 with the addition of Nancy N. Cain, MD, as consulting psychiatrist and Bonnie Kwiatkowski Kramer, PhD, serving as a consulting psychologist until she retired in 2018. Linda Quijano, MA, and Linda Matons, MA, served as behavioral specialists. Ms. Quijano succeeded Ms. Giesow as Director and stayed in that position until her retirement in 2018. Leadership of CI has transitioned to Kenneth Shamlian, PsyD, BCBA-D., who joined the faculty after postdoctoral training at the Munro Meyer Institute in Omaha.

One of the unique features of the CI program was the ability for providers to see consumers in their homes, schools, day programs, and other community settings, which greatly enhanced their ability to do effective assessments of behavioral challenges, provide staff and family training, and give other service recommendations. Initially the program served a wide range of children and adults, many of whom had been deinstitutionalized and were living in voluntary agency group homes. For the past 15 years, the program has served primarily people with IDD and ASD who live with their families.

## Mental Retardation and Developmental Disabilities (MRDD) Psychiatric Disorders Clinic

In 1985, Dr. Cain began to develop and coordinate training in IDD for Psychiatric fellows. When the C-MEDD program was funded, Dr. Cain developed relationships among the faculty of the other

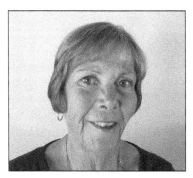

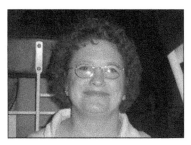

Figure 7.4. Bonnie Kramer, PhD. Photo from Dr. Kramer and reproduced with permission.

Figure 7.3. Virginia "Ginny" Giesow, MA. Photo from Ms. Giesow and reproduced with permission.

C-MEDD sites throughout the state, developed a curriculum, and set up sites both at URMC and in the community in which specialized psychiatric care training could take place. Since community outpatient psychiatric programs were very limited in the region, Dr. Cain established the MRDD Psychiatric Disorders Clinic (Davidson et al., 1999). The clinic focused on adults with IDD; the original clinic staff included Cain, two psychiatric nurse practitioners (Marilyn "Lyn" Sullivan, RN, MSN, and Mary Andolsek, RN, MSN), a

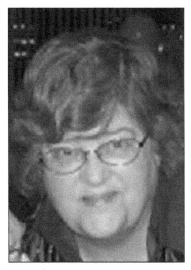

Figure 7.5. Linda Quijano, BS, MS. Photo from Ms. Quijano and reproduced with permission.

mental health social worker (Joanne Baxter, ACSW), and a consulting clinical/behavioral psychologist (Dr. Davidson). The clinic provided interdisciplinary diagnosis, individual and group psychotherapy, and community consultations. There was a close working relationship between the clinic and the CI Team.

Dr. Cain also developed a mobile team. The objective was to enrich the experience for the trainees as well as help provide skilled psychiatric consultations to community-based programs in the 17-county region. She and Gail Brownell, PhD, a behavioral psychologist from the FLDDSO, traveled to community-based programs to carry out comprehensive assessments and recommendations for care.

Once this framework was established, seminars were developed for the psychiatric residents (all of whom were required to rotate through the Clinic) and C-MEDD Fellows. They grew to include medical students (either as electives in the general medical curriculum or as part of their general psychiatric rotation); general pediatric residents; and master's-level nursing students. These students participated in the clinics and mobile unit teams as well.

This program improved the lives of numerous individuals with dual diagnoses, their families, and caregivers. The MRDD Psychiatric Disorders Clinic itself closed in 2004; but it spawned other similar programs in the region that are still in operation. In 2004, the American Psychiatric Association named Dr. Cain the recipient of the prestigious Frank Menaloscino, MD Award, recognizing an individual who has made significant contributions to psychiatric services, education, and research to persons with IDD.

## The Adult Offender Project

As a continuation of efforts to further work across systems and in the community, the SCDD applied for and received special funding in 1983 from the ADD. The funding was awarded to develop and implement cross system education and training for professionals in the Justice system. At the time, lack of cross-system training and outreach resulted in apprehension and confinement of anyone behaving atypically, so individuals with mental illness and with IDD were placed together and often treated similarly. Led by Ms. Messinger, the project promoted early identification of individuals with mental retardation and other disabilities and assisted justice professionals in dealing appropriately with these individuals, including diversion to alternatives to incarceration (Messinger et al., 1992). Margaret "Margie" McMahon, working with Ms. Messinger and James Clark, PhD, then director of the Monroe County Mental Health Clinic for Socio-Legal Services, worked to intercept alleged offenders when first apprehended and channel them to Dr. Clark's clinic for evaluation, while identifying necessary services both within the criminal justice system and in the IDD community to facilitate appropriate placement before cases reached the courts. Training was given to the judiciary, jailers, probation and parole officers, and staff of the Jail Ministry. Professionals from the developmental service system were placed in the county's Court Intake Clinic and in the Probation department. These individuals assisted in training, early identification, and, when appropriate, cross-system collaboration. The three-year project allowed for opportunities to discuss the project and disseminate information about it both within New York State and nationally.

## Program in Aging and Developmental Disabilities (PADD)

Between the 1950s and 1980s, trends in survival began to shift upwards. People with IDD were surviving into older age and the service delivery system was not prepared for this event. Moreover, predictive models suggested the trend would continue in a positively accelerated fashion for the foreseeable future. The ADD recognized this important trend and made Training Initiative Program (TIP) awards available to UCEDDs to enable them to address the demonstrable shortages in personnel with expertise in aging services. In 1986, following a site visit focused on whether to develop a program in aging, Jenny C. Overeynder, ACSW, PhD, was appointed to lead an effort to secure a TIP in Aging. The effort first involved a community-wide federally funded planning effort and culminated in TIP funding in 1987. Subsequently, SCDD collaborated with the Rose F. Kennedy Center in the Bronx, the Waisman Center in Madison, Wisconsin, and the Child Development Center at the University of Tennessee in Memphis to demonstrate in multiple sites the community-wide planning effort to plan for the needs of older adults with IDD. This collaboration was led by Ms. Burns and Dr. Sulkes.

The focus was training both community providers and preservice personnel drawn from the URMC's Center on Aging, and

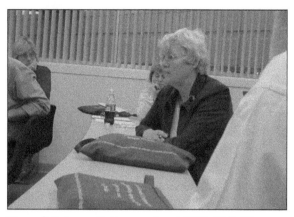

Figure 7.6. Jenny C. Overeynder, ACSW., PhD. Photo from SCDD archives and reproduced with permission.

other departments addressing adult health and requirements for specialized community services.

Plans to develop a Regional Center in Aging and Developmental Disabilities were implemented. This included infusion of content on this topic in existing courses on aging in a variety of colleges and universities, a PADD fellowship, development of training materials and many in-service education offerings, not only in the region, but statewide and nationally as well. The project established a close working relationship with Ronald Lucchino, PhD, a gerontologist at Utica College, Kathleen Bishop, PhD, a specialist in aging with IDD based in Rome, New York, and Richard Machemer, PhD, a biologist at St. John Fisher College in Rochester with an interest in gerontology. Later in the project's history, C. Michael Henderson, MD, joined as its first geriatrician. Dr. Henderson, who was trained in both internal medicine and pediatrics, had completed both a developmental pediatrics fellowship at SCDD and geriatrics fellowship at University of Rochester. Dr. Henderson contributed to teaching, service, and research prior to leaving the University of Rochester in 2009. A major contribution was his demonstration of specialized geriatric assessment for older adults with IDD, which he developed at the Monroe Community Hospital (Henderson et al., 2000). Laura M. Robinson, MPH, served as coordinator of PADD during this period. PADD continued until

2007 under the direction of Dr. Bishop, who assumed leadership after Dr. Overeynder retired.

## *Coordination of Care for Chronically Ill Children*

The complex multidisciplinary needs of children with chronic illnesses had been apparent for many years. Although managed care models for primary care were developing nationwide, children with special health care needs continued to

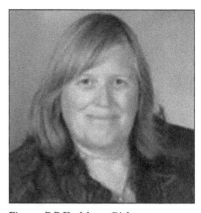

Figure 7.7 Kathleen Bishop, PhD. Photo from Dr. Bishop and reproduced with permission.

have high rates of hospitalization and their care was costly (Liptak et al., 1998; 1999). Ms. Burns led work to first engage the Monroe County Department of Health, and then Finger Lakes Blue Cross/ Blue Shield, to support a model of paying the Department of Pediatrics for services like social work and nutrition. Such services were not covered under regular fee-for-service insurance for children with a broad range of special health care needs.

Gregory S. Liptak, MD, MPH, played a major role in this project. He led the multidisciplinary clinical service that addressed the complex needs of children and youth with motor disabilities including cerebral palsy and spina bifida. His advocacy for this population led to the inclusion of spasticity management with Botox and baclofen pumps, inclusion of orthopedics and orthotics in the team care. His dual appointment and activities in general pediatrics was the precursor to what we today call Complex Care. For this work, Dr. Liptak received the Arnold J. Capute Award from the Council on Children with Disabilities of the American Academy of Pediatrics. Dr. Liptak left the University of Rochester in 2006 to lead the division of Developmental and Behavioral Pediatrics at Upstate Medical University in Syracuse. He died in 2012.

Dr. Liptak, Ms. Burns, and others performed an analysis that demonstrated that supporting such services resulted in substantial

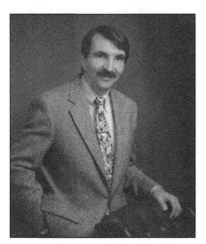

Figure 7.8. Gregory S. Liptak, MD, MPH. Photo from Dr. Liptak's family and reproduced with permission.

cost savings by keeping the children out of the hospital. Based on this evidence, ongoing coordination-of-care support from the local insurers was to continue for over a decade. These efforts occurred in the early 1980s when few benchmarks and guideposts existed. Ms. Burns was able to promote a clearly visionary collaboration between a university medical center, community providers, local government, third-party payers, and consumers. This effort, known then as the Coordination of Care for Chronically Ill Children (or CCCIC) project, was the precursor of other projects within the Department of Pediatrics. But the emphasis was to change to family-centered care.

## Physician Training Project

For coordinated care to work on behalf of families and children, provision of services and supports needed change. During the late 1970s parents took their children to the pediatrician general practitioner in one location, accessed other ancillary services in other locations, and had limited ability to engage in the process of developing an interdisciplinary plan of care and serve as a full member of the care delivery team. Change began with health care provider training. Ms. Burns led several training initiatives involving community-based physicians and dentists, as well as UCEDD trainees as early as 1980. Ms. Burns recruited several partners to help with this effort: Drs. William Kenney, Steve Sulkes, John Brooks, Richard Kreipe, Jorge Davila, and Stanley Novak, to mention a few.

## International Initiatives

In the mid-1980s, a few SCDD faculty members began to provide international technical assistance and outreach training. The first such initiative started in 1988 and took place as a part of the Partners of the Americas (PoA) chapter in Rochester, which partnered with Antigua-Barbuda in the eastern Caribbean. During that year, Drs. Davidson and Schworm visited the island nation and spent about one week providing individual assessments and consulting with staff members and administrators in several community-based children's services agencies. Some time was also spent consulting with Gwendolyn Tonge, the leader of the Antigua-Barbuda PoA chapter, and Hon. Reuben Harris, the Minister of Education. During 1990, Dr. Davidson returned to Antigua with James Mroczek, Executive Director of the Arc of Monroe County, with the objective of assisting the service system in developing employment services. This initiative was conducted with limited funding from the Rochester PoA chapter and the Government of Antigua-Barbuda. That same year, Ms. Barbara Charles of the Adele School for Handicapped Children, was an SCDD long-term trainee. The funding for the Antigua-Barbuda initiative ended in 1991.

In 1989, SCDD arranged for Drs. Davidson and Sulkes, and speech-language pathologist Edna Carter Young, PhD, to spend a week in Bermuda evaluating children with severe IDD at the Orange Valley School, providing in-service educational activities and consulting with government officials. This consultation was affectionately dubbed the Windjammer Mobile Unit by Dr. Sulkes. A series of follow-up discussions took place about one year later; and in 1991, Ms. Brenda Wilson, a speech language pathologist from Bermuda's Ministry of Education, was a long-term trainee at SCDD.

Although quite modest in scope, these two projects established a collective interest in international activities that formed the basis for much larger initiatives that took place later and also led to formulation of principles of such international collaboration on IDD projects (Davidson et al., 1992).

## Collaboration with NYS UCEDDs and the NYSDDPC

Apart from SCDD, New York State is home to two other federally funded UCEDDs: The Rose F. Kennedy Center at the Albert
Einstein College of Medicine in the Bronx and the Westchester
Institute for Human Development in Valhalla. The three UCEDDs
often collaborate on a variety of projects with statewide impact. An
additional, nonfederally funded program, the Developmental Disabilities Center at the St. Lukes–Roosevelt Hospital Center in Manhattan sometimes joined these collaborations. Many projects were
accomplished in collaboration with the NYSDDPC. Some examples of collaborative projects include statewide needs assessments,
statewide technical assistance, preparation of technical reports for
the NYSDDPC, and provision of community-based training activities. The four program directors (Dr. Davidson, Herbert J. Cohen,
MD, at the Rose Kennedy Center, Ansley Bacon, PhD, at Valhalla,
and Louis Cooper, MD, and Philip Ziring, MD, in Manhattan) all
knew each other very well and were good friends, leading to very
productive and fruitful projects. All are now retired; but collaborations continue.

# INTERLUDE
# (OR LET US TAKE A
# BREAK FROM ACRONYMS)

We are about halfway through our story. You have been bombarded with acronyms. After a reading of an early version of the manuscript, one of our coauthors remarked: "My head is spinning with all the acronyms! You need a glossary." Well, we included a list of abbreviations; but that did not seem enough remedy for a problem that plagues all organizations.

We have written about Stephen B. Sulkes, MD. You know from our narrative he has had a major impact on training and service programs. But you may not know that he is also a fine poet and lyricist. He has composed many alternative lyrics to famous melodies. He has done so both in Rochester, at AUCD (oops, we hope you will forgive the mention of an acronym), and at other venues and organizations around the world. We are not sure if he has ever been compensated for his work.

The first author used to cringe whenever Dr. Sulkes led our group in song. Dr. Davidson now admits his mistake. Dr. Sulkes' lyrics brought cheer and laughter to any group where they were performed. I really was not then and am not now a grump; and at some level, both Susan and I appreciated what Steve was contributing.

Over the many years Dr. Sulkes has been with the University of Rochester, he must have composed dozens of alternative lyrics. We are sure none were ever published—not until now. We asked Dr. Sulkes to pick one of his poems for inclusion in this book. Appropriately, he picked one that makes fun of all the acronyms accumulated at the center, at least until the mid-1990s. We deserve no less!

Identity Crisis
Stephen B. Sulkes, MD

When I first came to work here it was at DCDD
And now and then I saw a kid cared for by BDC.
We lacked coordination and a funder with a name
But then we got the things we sought and this is how they came:
Andrew J. Kirch Developmental Services Center—If you want to
say this name you need a fulltime mentor,
But if you keep on using it, you'll cheer for its inventor.
Andrew J. Kirch Developmental Services Center!
After a while my clinic's name was changed to CDA.
And Easter Seals took over and my comment was "Hooray!"
The whole division couldn't buck this trend for very long
So even sans endowment we were named for Sandy Strong.
Andrew J. Kirch Developmental Services Center—
If you want to say this name you need a fulltime mentor,
But if you keep on using it, you'll cheer for its inventor.
Andrew J. Kirch Developmental Services Center!
You all have heard the saying that is used throughout the city
That a camel is a horse that was designed by a committee.
You may think it's a great idea or that it is a shame,
But love it or revile it, that is how we got this name:
Andrew J. Kirch Developmental Services Center—
If you want to say this name you need a fulltime mentor,
But if you keep on using it, you'll cheer for its inventor.
Andrew J. Kirch Developmental Services Center!
So now we have a brand-new name to keep 'til we go under.
It proves we are responsive to the whims of every funder.
We say: Go forth and diagnose!
Coordinate!
Be vital!
Until the university decides to change our title!
Andrew J. Kirch Developmental Services Center—
If you want to say this name you need a fulltime mentor,
But if you keep on using it, you'll cheer for its inventor.
Andrew J. Kirch Developmental Services Center!

*[Note to reader: Any rhythmic similarity to known show tunes is purely
purposeful. SBS]*

# Chapter Eight

# EXPANSION

*Everyone wants to live on top of the mountain, but all the happiness and growth occurs while you're climbing it.*
—Andy Rooney

Now back to work.

As of 1990, the SCDD interdisciplinary team included sixty-four faculty and technical staff, representing 14 academic disciplines from the University of Rochester and seven other higher learning institutions in upstate New York. Consumer services were provided to 1,585 people in that year, 5,434 community-based personnel received outreach training sponsored by SCDD, and faculty and students published a total of 23 peer-reviewed papers or chapters. The 1990 income was $1,685,707. Over the next 15 years, the income would increase to over $5 million due to growth in research programs, new training initiatives, and the expansion of clinical services.

Further growth of SCDD was linked to developing discretionary funding. For its first 15 years, SCDD funding was limited to grants and contracts for specific programs; income from clinical services rarely reached a break-even point. In the mid 1990s the Department of Pediatrics designated the emerging program in Autism Spectrum Disorders as one of its strategic targets for growth, which freed discretionary funding for new faculty positions. Beginning in the late 1990s several recruitments took place that brought new key personnel to SCDD's faculty. There was also an effort to raise the level of gift and bequeathal funding specific to IDD. Several key gifts were received, including multiyear funding from the Andrew J. Kirch Charitable Trust and gifts from individual donors.

By 1990 long-range plans for SCDD reflected emergent major themes, largely guided by UCEDD federal requirements. Growth after 1990 was driven by the changing landscape for research and clinical funding regionally, nationally, and internationally. Deinstitutionalization had been nearly completed, at least in New York State. Large aggregate care settings were replaced with community-based small group or individual residential alternatives. The shift from a focus on only children to a concern for age-span services and supports in SCDD was now complete. The SCDD training program had matured sufficiently to support more ambitious initiatives both within the UR and in the community. Service and training also were impacted dramatically by the appearance of larger and larger numbers of consumers with suspected Autism Spectrum Disorders. Recruitment of new faculty with help from the Department of Pediatrics Strategic Plan funds, in turn brought a much larger focus on research.

## New Recruitments

Between 1994 and 2001, SCDD was successful in recruiting early to mid-career faculty members who collectively would go on to shape the future direction of developmental behavioral pediatrics at URMC. Susan L. Hyman, MD, joined the faculty in 1994. Dr. Hyman completed a Developmental Pediatrics fellowship with Arnold J. Capute, MD, MPH, and Mark Batshaw, MD, PhD, of the Kennedy-Krieger Institute at Johns Hopkins University School of Medicine. She brought a special interest in autism spectrum disorders, going on to develop a very fruitful collaboration with Patricia Rodier, PhD, an embryologist in the Department of Obstetrics and Gynecology, about which more will be said further on. Dr. Hyman has had a long and distinguished career in Developmental and Behavioral Pediatrics, both at URMC and around the world, for which she has been recognized by receiving the Arnold J. Capute Award.

Karin Theurer-Kaufman, PhD, a State of New York University at Stony Brook–trained behavioral analyst, also joined the faculty following completion of a pediatric psychology fellowship with Dr. Davidson. She led the first clinical program focused on community consultation around Autism Spectrum Disorders (ASD) in SCDD. Dr. Theurer-Kaufman in turn recruited Caroline Magyar, PhD, who succeeded her as program director, and Tristram Smith, PhD, who had trained at UCLA with Ivar Lovaas, PhD Dr. Smith was an expert in intensive behavioral interventions for children with ASD. His career at URMC eventually led to many NIH research grant awards that were informed by the collaboration of academic clinicians in community sites. In 2002, Daniel Mruzek, PhD, who had trained with Henry Leland, PhD, at the Nisonger Center, Ohio State University's UCEDD, and who had a special interest in adaptive behavior, joined the team. He was followed in 2002–3 by Deborah Napolitano, PhD, David McAdam, PhD, and Dennis Mozingo, PhD, all behavioral analysts. Finally, Jennifer Zarcone, PhD, joined SCDD in 2004. Drs. Napolitano and McAdam had trained with Stephen Schroeder, PhD, at the Shiefelbusch Center, Kansas University, which focused on application of behavioral interventions for individuals with IDD. Dr. Zarcone, who earned her PhD at the University of Florida, went first to The Kennedy-Krieger Institute where she completed a postdoctoral fellowship and remained

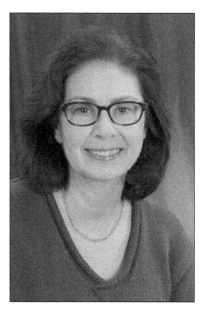

Figure 8.1. Susan L. Hyman, MD.

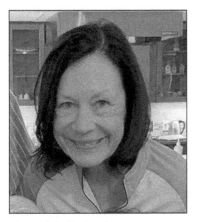

Figure 8.2. Karin Theurer-Kaufman, PhD. Photo from Dr. Theurer-Kaufman and reproduced with permission.

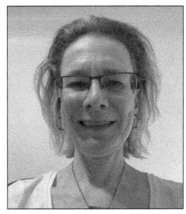

Figure 8.3. Caroline Magyar, PhD. Reproduced with permission.

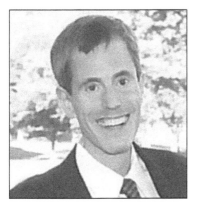

Figure 8.4. Tristram Harry Smith, PhD. Photo obtained from Susan Hyman, MD, and reproduced with permission from Jennifer Katz, PhD.

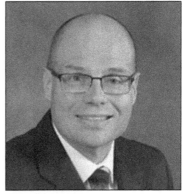

Figure 8.5. Danial Mruzek, PhD. Reproduced with permission.

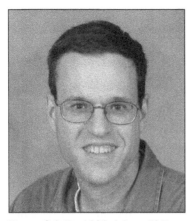

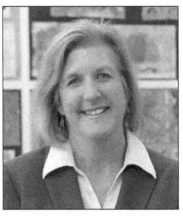

Figure 8.6. David McAdam, PhD. Photo from Dr. McAdam and reproduced with permission.

Figure 8.7. Jennifer Zarcone, PhD. Reproduced with permission.

three more years on the faculty before going to Kansas where she worked with Drs. Schroeder and Travis Thompson, PhD. She came to Rochester from the Shiefelbusch Center.

## Leadership Education in Neurodevelopmental and Related Disabilities

As noted earlier, at the time the original legislation providing funding for UCEDDs was authorized, Congress created several programs to support postgraduate training in IDD. One of them, now known as Leadership Education in Neurodevelopmental Disabilities (LEND) was and still is administered by MCHB within the Health Resources and Services Administration (HRSA), US Department of Health and Human Services. Until 1992, the program was limited to about 20 UCEDDs. By the early 1990s the UCEDD network began to rapidly expand and pressure was brought to bear on MCHB to expand the LEND program. Congress authorized such an expansion in 1992 and SCDD prepared an application for newly appropriated funds. The application was approved and funded in 1994 with Dr. Sulkes as the program director, and with

Ms. Burns serving as associate director. Awarding of this grant was a watershed moment for SCDD since it provided stipends for long-term trainees and training support faculty representing 10 clinical disciplines. From its inception, the LEND program graduated around 10 long-term trainees and over 40 shorter term trainees annually. Since graduate training in several of these disciplines was not available at University of Rochester, this provided an opportunity for fresh collaborations with other colleges and universities in western New York, including State of New York College at Geneseo, State University of New York College at Brockport, State University of New York University at Buffalo, Cornell University, and Nazareth College of Rochester.

Table 8.1 shows the growth of interdisciplinary preservice training at SCDD, which can be attributed to the LEND Program. Between 1997 and 2018, 1,299 preservice trainees were enrolled in SCDD preservice training activities, with about 75% spending 150 or more contact hours per year in clinical, research, or other educational settings. In other words, in the 12 years preceding 1997 reviewed earlier, most SCDD trainees were short term. In the years following 1997, trainee contact hours had shifted to mostly long term. Table 8.1 also shows that the distribution of trainees by discipline had become much broader compared to the data we describe for 1985 to 1997.

## Clinical Disciplines and the Special Role of Nursing

By 1990, SCDD, including LEND had expanded to include 13 clinical disciplines. Each discipline contributed to SCDD's overall growth, both in terms of service and support capacity, education, and research. Nursing played an especially important role because of the program focus on health promotion and health-care delivery Nurses became a part of SCDD with its merger with the Birth Defects Center: The first BDC nurse, Sharon Bidwell Cerone, RN, MSN, PhD, served as the first nursing discipline coordinator. Advanced practice nurses were integrated with developmental diagnostic services and became an important component of the SCDD training program. The link between SCDD and the School of Nursing became stronger and pediatric and adult psychiatric nurse

Table 8.1. Preservice Education Trainees at DBP 1997–2018.

| Discipline or Major | ≥ 9 Contact Hours Per Year | ≥150 Contact Hours per Year |
|---|---|---|
| Audiology | 15 | 15 |
| Biological Sciences | 4 | 2 |
| Dentistry | 22 | 10 |
| Disability Studies | 3 | 0 |
| Education | 46 | 30 |
| Epidemiology | 3 | 2 |
| Family Studies | 1 | 1 |
| Advocates | 7 | 7 |
| Genetics/Genetic Counseling | 2 | 2 |
| Human Development | 8 | 2 |
| Interdisciplinary Majors | 31 | 0 |
| General Studies | 1 | 0 |
| Medicine | 525 | 437 |
| Mental/Behavioral Health | 2 | 0 |
| Nursing | 39 | 22 |
| Nutrition | 37 | 7 |
| Occupational Therapy | 14 | 10 |
| Physical Therapy | 32 | 30 |
| Psychiatry | 18 | 2 |
| Psychology | 140 | 85 |
| Public Health | 54 | 29 |
| Social Work | 40 | 46 |
| Communication Disorders | 31 | 29 |
| Other | 184 | 133 |
| TOTALS | 1299 | 908 |

practitioners joined the SCDD faculty. Dr. Bidwell Cerone left LEND in the mid-1980s and was replaced first by Barbara Masiulis, RN, MS, then by Alison Schultz, RN, MS, EdD, and Jane Tuttle, RN, PhD. As noted, with the increased demand for services and limited number of board-certified Developmental Behavioral pediatricians, the clinical service has trained and incorporated a total of nine pediatric nurse practitioners in all clinical service lines.

## Andrew J. Kirch Developmental Services Center

Although consolidation of clinical services and supports was accomplished during the 1980s, the SCDD's various clinics continued to operate as independent columns within the whole. A series of events beginning in 1995 influenced this situation. Until that point the Physical Disabilities clinical program (formally known as the Birth Defects Center and then the Easter Seals Physical Disabilities Program) was partially funded by the Easter Seals Foundation. This funding stream came to an end in the early 1990s. By 1995, financing had become a threat to continuation of this program, despite the high quality of its clinical services and advocacy, the commitment of the interdisciplinary staff, and most of all, the caring and focused leadership of Dr. Liptak, who was universally admired by his staff and consumers. A series of discussions took place between Henra Briskin, ACSW (the SCDD Social Worker working in the Easter Seals Physical Disabilities Program) and James Vazzana, Esq. (a Rochester attorney whose law firm was the executor of the Andrew J. Kirch Charitable Trust) that led to a commitment from the Charitable Trust to provide substantial deficit-reduction funding to SCDD in order to maintain and expand services to children with physical disabilities. In 1997, SCDD received permission to name its entire clinical services component after Andrew J. Kirch (who was a prominent Rochester automobile dealer). At the same time, changes in local health care financing and reimbursement began to exert pressure on providers to simplify access for consumers, and reduce costs though providing more efficient models of care.

The Kirch Charitable Trust provided additional support to SCDD to fund an annual Pediatric Grand Rounds. Among the

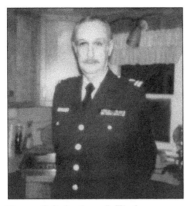

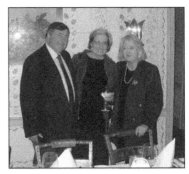

Figure 8.8. Andrew J. Kirsh. Photo from James Vazzana and reproduced with permission.

Figure 8.9. *From left:* James Vazzana, Esq. (executor, AJ Kirsh Charitable Trust), Randi Hagerman MD (Kirch Visiting Professor), Patricia Vazzana (trustee, AJ Kirch Charitable Trust). From SCDD archives and reproduced with permission from Mr. Vazzana.

distinguished speakers that came to Rochester between 2004 and 2010 were Randi Hagerman, MD (University of California at Davis), Dennis Harper, PhD (University of Iowa), Marilee Allen, MD (Johns Hopkins University), Karin B. Nelson, MD (NIH), and Marshalyn Yeargain Allsopp, MD (Centers for Disease Control and Prevention).

The relationship between SCDD and the Kirch Charitable Trust was a driving force that resulted in a major reorganization of the newly named Andrew J. Kirch Developmental Services Center to encompass a wider array of diagnostic and intervention options, improved one-stop care for consumers and their families, and a consolidation of duplicative administrative procedures that had existed prior to 1995. The Charitable Trust continued its generous support to SCDD for 21 years until it was dissolved in 2019.

## ASD Program and the
## Community Consultation Program (CCP)

In the early 1990s, the Rochester community began to identify a dramatic number of children with phenotypic signs and symptoms of ASD. This trend mirrored similar increases all over the world. Some of these children were referred for evaluations through the Kirch Center, but SCDD lacked clinical capacity, not just to provide a diagnosis, but more importantly, to respond to the growing need for home-based and school-based interventions. In 1994, SCDD embarked on implementing an intervention program for ASD under the leadership of Ms. Burns and Dr. Theurer-Kaufman. To meet the new demand for services and supports, a number of new faculty members with behavior analytic skills were hired (Drs. Mruzek, Magyar, Napolitano, McAdam, Mozingo, Smith, and Zarcone), financed largely by the development of contracts with school districts for consultation. ASD evaluations soon grew to account for the majority of Kirch Center diagnostic services annually; but it also spurred the development of the CCP, which provided outreach training and individual interventions to schools and families throughout the region; the CCP continued to grow larger and larger and eventually expanded to include consultations on behalf of children with any developmental diagnoses. The CCP built a novel model of technical assistance and program development for schools and agencies throughout Western New York using evidence-based behavioral approaches. Leadership of the CCP was assumed by Dr. Magyar when Dr. Theurer-Kaufman left SCDD in 1998, followed by Dr. Zarcone, then Dr. Mozingo, then Dr. McAdam until 2019.

ASD services and supports had a transformative influence on the future of SCDD. First, SCDD had recruited a large enough cadre of experts in ASD to assume a position of regional clinical leadership. Most consequential was its influence on school districts and BOCES programs as they began to develop more efficient ways to provide inclusive services and supports. Second, the skill sets of SCDD faculty recruited to the ASD Program extended from clinical service to training to research. Consequently, there was an increase in activity in all three of these domains, including increased research productivity, advances in model community services, new educational programs (including certification curricula in Applied Behavior Analysis in collaboration with the Warner Graduate School of Education and Human Development), and partnerships with community planning entities to prepare for the heretofore unanticipated growth in needs for expanded services and supports. With hundreds of new referrals, SCDD also developed new research projects that ultimately led to successful acquisition of state, federal, and private foundation funding. Finally, and probably most important, the growing awareness of ASD in the community played an important role in elevating the profile of SCDD within the University of Rochester, and ultimately leading to philanthropic activity that no one could have imagined only a few years earlier.

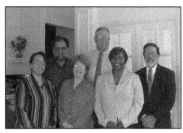

Figure 8.10. Klarberg Scholars 2005. *Front row,* Melanie Melendez (trainee), Dr. Hetherington, Wanda Nelomes (trainee) Dr. Davidson. *Back row,* Dr. Ciaizza, Mr. Klarberg. Reproduced with permission from Mr. Klarberg.

During this period, a small but significant project was started to promote an increase in representation in the IDD workforce of people of ethnic and cultural minority backgrounds. Joseph E. Klarberg, an investment advisor and friend of Dr. Davidson's, and his spouse, Judy, established the Elizabeth Klarberg Minority Scholars Program. The program was named after the Klarberg's older daughter, who had completed a summer internship at SCDD. Between 1995 and 2002 the program offered a scholarship for a summer placement at SCDD for one student per year from the Human Services department at the Monroe Community College, chaired by Professor Anthony Caiazza. In 2003, the placement was expanded to a duration of one semester. Dr. Hetherington coordinated the project.

# Chapter Nine

# EMERGENCE OF RESEARCH PROGRAMS

*I am convinced that an important stage of human thought will have been reached when the physiological and the psychological, the objective and the subjective, are actually united, when the tormenting conflicts or contradictions between my consciousness and my body will have been factually resolved or discarded.*

— Ivan Pavlov, 1932, pp. 93–94

During the 1990s and early 2000s, several research themes emerged, and resulted in substantial extramural funding.

## Mercury and Child Development

In the 1950s, mass poisonings took place in Minamata and Niigata, Japan. Hundreds of people died after consuming fish contaminated by industrial runoff containing methylmercury (Harada, 1968). Children born to pregnant women who were exposed to the toxic effluent were born with severe IDD. About 10 years later, another poisoning took place in Iraq, also involving methylmercury exposure; but in Iraq the exposure was from seed grain coated with a fungicide containing methylmercury (Amin-Zaki et al., 1974). After the Iraq outbreak, a team of investigators from the University of Rochester led by Thomas W. Clarkson, PhD, and including neurologists David Marsh, MD, and Dr. Myers, evaluated prenatally exposed Iraqi children and published data suggesting that intellectual and developmental abnormalities could result from exposure to methylmercury in the range that could be achieved by consuming ocean fish. Drs. Clarkson, Marsh, and Myers, together with Conrad F. Shamlaye, MD, MPH, MEcon, from the Ministry of Health in the Republic

of Seychelles initiated the Seychelles Child Development Study
(SCDS) in 1985 to test the hypothesis that prenatal exposure to
organic methylmercury (MeHg) from fish consumption could
lead to adverse neurodevelopmental outcomes in the offspring
of mothers who consumed fish. Dr. Davidson joined the study
team in 1990 and succeeded Dr. Clarkson as Principal Investigator in 2006. The evidence amassed during the over 30-year
duration of the SCDS has not supported the original hypothesis;
the studies have demonstrated that the pathway between MeHg
exposure and outcome is very complex and affected by nutrients
in fish and genetic factors. The likely story is that potential methylmercury neurotoxicity is modified by antioxidants and anti-
inflammatory compounds found in a diet high in fish (Davidson
et al., 1998; Davidson et al., 2008a; Myers et al., 2003; Strain et al.,
2008). These results have led to much public policy discussion
regarding fish consumption advisories issued by governments
around the world (Kaiser, 1996). Studies are underway to examine the influence of polymorphisms associated with genes that
regulate both nutrient metabolism and methylmercury transport
and clearance in both humans and *drosophila* (Llop et al., 2017;
Vorojeikina et al., 2017). In addition to organic mercury exposure from fish consumption, inorganic Hg exposure occurs from
dental amalgam fillings. Another line of inquiry, led by Gene
Watson, DDS, PhD, has focused on associations between child
development and the number of dental amalgam fillings in pregnant mothers and in children (Watson et al., 2011; 2013). Since
its inception, the SCDS has been continuously funded by multiple NIH research grants. The SCDS has also studied the effects of
methylmercury exposure on the auditory system, the heart, and
the immune system. Links between methylmercury exposure and
ASD have also been studied.

Assessing the developmental impacts of neurotoxic exposures
can be very difficult, especially when the study methodology is
the cohort study. For this reason, Dr. Davidson collaborated with
the late Bernard Weiss, PhD, and other SCDS team members to
develop and validate a comprehensive neurocognitive assessment
battery. The battery is called the Rochester Battery and serves as
a basis for examinations of the SCDS cohorts from 2006 onward
(Davidson et al., 2006).

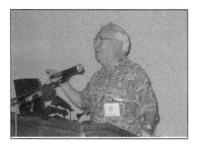

Figure 9.1. Thomas W. Clarkson, PhD. Reproduced with permission.

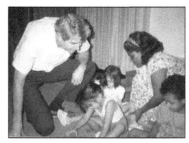

Figure 9.2. Gary J. Myers, MD (with Madam Choisy) examining Seychellois toddlers, circa 1989. Photo from SCDD archives and reproduced with permission.

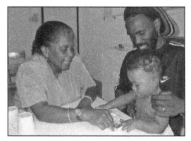

Figure 9.3. Octavie Choisy (long-serving study coordinator of the Seychelles Child Development Study) administering a neurodevelopmental test.

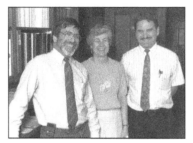

Figurer 9.4. Basil Porter, MBBCh, MPH (R), with Drs. Davidson and Cain. Photo from SCDD archives and reproduced with permission.

In addition to Drs. Myers and Davidson, many current and former SCDD faculty and staff have been a part of the SCDS, including Drs. Smith and Mruzek, Mark Orlando, PhD, Ms. Burns, Kelley Yost, PhD, Edna Carter-Young, PhD, Donna Palumbo, PhD, Jean Reeves, MS, Lisa Rodgers, and Catherine Imhof.

Dr. Davidson remained solo PI of the SCDS until 2013. He and Edwin vanWijngaarden, MPH, PhD, an environmental epidemiologist in the Department of Public Health Science, then shared leadership until 2018, when Dr. Davidson fully retired.

## Health and Mental Health Status among Adults and Older Adults with IDD

As the MRDD Psychiatric Disorders Program became an integral part of the community with more and more complex individuals being referred a research component was added. A wealth of knowledge was gained in both ways to diagnose and ways to treat individuals with dual diagnoses. Useful models were also emerged that might be replicated in other communities.

With funds from the US Department of Health and Human Services, they also explored ways to set up a similar program in Israel. The project was based in Beer Sheva, Israel, at the Ben Gurion University of the Negev.

Dr. Davidson also led epidemiological research on health and mental health characteristics of older persons with IDD. He partnered with Matthew P. Janicki, PhD, coordinator of Aging Services for NYS OPWDD. The project was responsible for the development of the Rochester Health Status Survey (Davidson et al., 2008b). Once validated, the RHSS and its subsequent revisions were then used as a data collection tool for studies that followed. The project eventually led to a further partnership with the University of Illinois at Chicago's Rehabilitation Research and Training Center on Aging with Intellectual Disabilities, directed by Tamar Heller, PhD. It also led to two major meetings, one in Geneva sponsored by the World Health Organization and the other in Tampa, Florida, at the University of South Florida sponsored by NIH. These conferences yielded three books and a special issue of the *Journal of Policy and Practice in Intellectual Disabilities* (Davidson et al., 2004). The project continues today under the leadership of Robert Fortuna, MD, MPH.

## ASD Research

The initial collaborative relationship between Drs. Hyman and Rodier was focused on a study of behavioral and early genetic factors related to ASD. In 1997, Dr. Rodier was awarded one of the first six NIH center grants for ASD research, the Collaborative Programs for Excellence in Autism (CPEA); Dr. Hyman was

a coinvestigator. The Rochester CPEA focuses on studying
brainstem development and
the role of early developmental genes in the pathophysi-
ology of autism. In 2003, Dr.
Rodier successfully competed
for a multiproject center
grant to establish a STAART
program (Studies to Advance
Autism Research and Treatment) at URMC, with Dr.
Hyman as co-PI and Drs.
Magyar and Smith as coin-

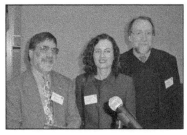

Figure 9.5. Tamar Heller, PhD,
and Matthew P. Janicki, PhD, with
Dr. Davidson. Photo from SCDD
archives and reproduced with
permission.

vestigators. The NIH made only 11 such awards. Dr. Magyar led
the Facility Core that engaged in phenotyping participants. The
three research projects funded included a double blind placebo
controlled challenge study examining the behavioral effect of
ingesting gluten, casein, or the combination compared to placebo
in children with autism (led by Dr. Hyman); a study examining
facial movement and expression in children with and without
autism (led by Loisa Bennetto, PhD, of the Department of Clinical and Social Psychology), and a study of the effect of community
administered Early Intense Behavioral Intervention in preschool
age children with autism compared to treatment as usual (led by
Dr. Smith). In 2008, Drs. Hyman and Smith successfully competed
to become a part of a newly formed coalition in North America
known as the Autism Speaks Autism Treatment Network (AS
ATN), which created the opportunity for additional research funding. The STAART program Assessment Core evaluated children
for inclusion in STAART research programs, the AS ATN Database
collected clinical information on phenotype and medical and
behavioral care to inform a growing literature on co-occurring
conditions with ASD. Later, a divisional research data base was
developed that allowed families who were seen in the clinical setting to learn about research projects that might be appropriate
for their child.

Dr. Smith successfully competed for several NIH individual
investigator awards (R01s). The total of effort devoted to these

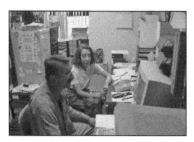

Figure 9.6. Patricia Rodier, PhD with Dr. Liptak.

projects created a thriving interdepartmental research community that included SCDD, Dr. Rodier's laboratory, and a group of investigators from the Department of Clinical and Social Psychology led by Dr. Bennetto. The STAART project was completed in 2009, but research efforts continued with increasing vigor thereafter. Other faculty secured funding for their research, including Drs. Mruzek, McAdam, Silverman, and Iadarola. Consequently, the Rochester ASD research group grew and garnered international prominence. The research portfolio focusing on behavioral interventions and evaluation of communication and gesture formed the basis for a viable translational research program that continues into the present.

## Behavioral Science Facility Core

In 2010 SCDD partnered with the Department of Environmental Medicine's Environmental Health Research Center to institute research quality behavioral assessment protocols for animal and human research studies taking place at URMC. The facility core's mission was "to advance the field of behavioral science by providing high quality services to scientists performing behavioral studies" (URMC website). The service had two interactive components, one for animal research headed by Dr. Deborah Cory-Slechta and the other for human research, directed by Dr. Zarcone until she left the URMC. The human studies component was then directed by Dr. Mruzek in collaboration with Erica Augustine, MD, of the Department of Neurology.

## A First Attempt at Organizing a Mental Retardation and Developmental Disabilities Research Center

In 1997 Drs. Davidson and Liptak began efforts to create a Center for Research on Mental Retardation and Developmental Disabilities. The goal was to submit a proposal to NICHD for a Mental Retardation and Developmental Disabilities Research Center (MRDDRC) in 2002. By 1998, a seminar series was begun, funding was approved from the Dean's Office to support a small grants program, and a proposal to plan the project was submitted to the Joseph P. Kennedy Foundation (but ultimately not funded). There was a lot of local interest in this project. But at the time, NICHD required applicants to have significant grant support from that agency's MRDD branch, which Rochester did not have. This requirement was modified in later years, which would facilitate efforts to organize an application for MRDDRC funding later. The project ended in 2002, after the NICHD director, Duane Alexander, MD, visited Rochester and encouraged a focus on ASD research, which was growing rapidly under the leadership of Drs. Hyman and Rodier.

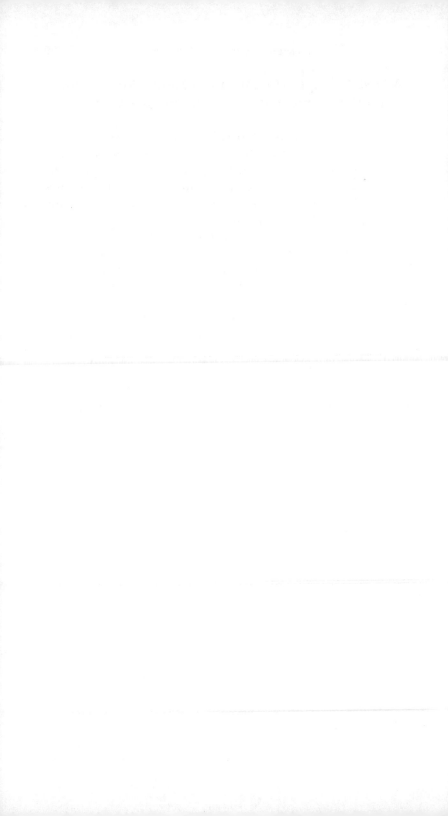

# Chapter Ten

# CHANGE IN THE WIND

*If there is no struggle, there is no progress.*
—Frederick Douglass

*I can honestly say that I was never affected by the question of the
success of an undertaking. If I felt it was the right thing to do, I
was for it regardless of the possible outcome.*
—Golda Meir

By 2006, SCDD had grown from a very small clinical program
within the Department of Pediatrics to a multifaceted inter-
collegiate center with international partners and significant local,
regional, national, and international impact. Its programs had
been expanded to include services and supports, interdisciplinary
training, and both basic and clinical research. Yet transformational
growth was still to come.

In 2006, after 30 years of directing SCDD and 25 years as Division Chief, Dr. Davidson stepped aside to assume leadership of the
Seychelles Child Development Study and pursue other research
goals. At the same time as Dr. Davidson moved away from SCDD
leadership, Christine Burns stepped aside as Associate Division
Chief to assume pediatric department responsibilities and to
work on coordination of care projects at the departmental level
until her untimely death in 2016. Dr. Sulkes assumed responsibility for directing the UCEDD in 2007. This appointment assured
federal funders of leadership continuity, an important issue since
the UCEDD competing renewal application was due in 2008. It
was renewed in 2009. Soon thereafter, Dr. Hetherington became
UCEDD codirector; and in 2014 she took over as UCEDD Director. Dr. Sulkes remained as UCEDD Co-Director and director of
the LEND program until 2019.

After a year of interim leadership by Nina Schor, MD, PhD, the newly arrived chair of Pediatrics a Child Neurologist, Dr. Hyman was appointed to succeed Dr. Davidson as Division Chief. Prior to her appointment as Chief, Dr. Hyman negotiated a change in the administrative structure of the Division to include a focus in both developmental and behavioral pediatrics. It was renamed the Division of Neurodevelopmental and Behavioral Pediatrics (NDBP) and became the academic home of the UCEDD (still named SCDD). SCDD remained a major administrative component of NDBP and was responsible for advocacy programs and many community-based activities. This was a big change for everyone concerned; it took some time to work out the management details. The redesignation of the Division as one that provided an academic and clinical home to both developmental and behavioral pediatrics had roots extending to the very beginning of its history although divisional culture evolved from a very strong focus on IDD. Many faculty and staff had and continued to have academic and functional roles related to the UCEDD, which in turn provided both direction to their work and core and administrative funding to support it.

Several factors influenced change in the divisional culture. First, Dr. Hyman came from a background in both developmental and behavioral pediatrics. If these two strains were to effectively come together and be integrated into a new focus for the division, Dr. Hyman was well-suited to oversee it.

The second factor influencing change was the increasing impact of ASD. Many children and young adults with ASD sought clinical services related to behavioral disorders. The divisional clinical service's historical approaches to providing developmental diagnoses did not include treatment of behavioral disorders; so clinical services to address the need were developed. In turn, community donors began to recognize the importance of these programs though large gifts. Ties were developed with the William and Mildred Levine Foundation that eventuated in the building of a dedicated clinic whose physical space was welcoming to individuals with sensory, motor, and cognitive needs. We will discuss these initiatives further on. Also, funding for clinical and translational research addressing early intensive behavioral therapy continued to increase, which required more commitment of institutional space for DBP. Research space was assigned in the newly constructed Saunders Research Building. Greater focus on developmental and behavioral pediatrics such as never seen before ensued from the Department of Pediatric and Medical Center administrations. Dr. Schor, the chairperson of Pediatrics, as a child neurologist understood the importance of biopsychosocial medicine for people with ASD and IDD.

The impact of the increased awareness of ASD and increasing prevalence rates nationally and locally on the divisional culture was profound. More faculty and staff with backgrounds in ASD were hired and began to interact with existing divisional faculty and staff. The awarding of the AS ATN by Autism Speaks to Drs. Hyman and Smith in 2008 (Lynn Cole, MSN, PNP, became the third co-Principal Investigator) allowed the clinical, research, and advocacy aspects of autism practice at the University of Rochester to achieve national stature. The AS ATN was focused on establishing a standard of care for diagnosis and management of children and youth with ASD in partnership with families and self-advocates. It led to Family Navigation in the clinical setting and an increased role for families in clinical and research planning and improvement.

ASD research across the university became an important part of the University of Rochester strategic Plan in 2014 and IDD became a part of the Department of Pediatrics Strategic plan with the arrival of Dr. Patrick Brophy as the 8th Chair of Pediatrics in 2017. This was fueled by the interest of B. Thomas Golisano, the principal benefactor of the Children's Hospital, in care for individuals with IDD across the lifespan and the recruitment of John Foxe, PhD, a neuroscientist and codirector of the IDDRC at the Albert Einstein College of Medicine. Dr. Foxe was named Professor and Killian J. and Caroline F. Schmitt chair of the Department of Neuroscience and director of the E. J. Del Monte Neuroscience Institute. He was also charged with bringing an IDDRC to URMC. By the early 2000s, funded research addressing both molecular and clinical questions in IDD had reached a critical mass and Medical Center Administration recognized the time was right to apply for an IDDRC. NDBP was to play a key role in this effort with Dr. Tristram Smith named as codirector. His death in August 2018 left a void in the IDDRC planning filled by Jonathan Mink,

MD, PhD, of child neurology. The grant proposal was submitted to the National Institutes of Health in January 2020. Just as we go to press with this book, Drs. Foxe and Mink were notified by NIH that the Rochester IDDRC proposal was funded. When combined with UCEDD and LEND grants already in place, the IDDRC places URMC among the small group of Universities with all three top-tier programs in IDD.

It took a lot of networking, leadership at the national level, and local media activities for the excellence of NDBP ASD efforts to be recognized. It was astonishing to see the rise of the profile of NDBP.

A third factor that affected change was divisional stewardship of the legacy of Drs. Haggerty and Friedman at the University of Rochester. The acknowledgment of the importance of the bio-psychosocial impact on child development for children with and without developmental disabilities is an important component of the medical and graduate education provided by NDBP faculty. In addition, it incorporated the goals of the *Haggerty-Friedman Psychosocial Fund for Developmental and Behavioral Pediatrics*. Drs. Haggerty and Friedman created this fund in 1993 through a bequeathal to pass to the Department of Pediatrics upon their deaths. Their intent was to establish a Division of Behavioral Pediatrics. Some funds were made available immediately to establish the Haggerty-Friedman Psychosocial Fund for Studies in Developmental-Behavioral Pediatrics. Dr. Davidson followed by Christine Burns and Dr. Richard Kreipe (then chief of Adolescent Medicine) coordinated the project from 1994 until 2008. Dr. Hyman assumed this responsibility in 2008, when the administrative home for the project was changed from the Department of Pediatrics to NDBP. The principal function of the project included small research grants to young investigators, promotion of education in developmental and behavioral pediatrics for pediatric residents and for medical students, and an annual Haggerty-Friedman Pediatric Grand Rounds. The annual Grand Rounds brought many well-known speakers to Rochester, including Laurie Bauman, PhD (Albert Einstein College of Medicine), Beth Ellen Davis, MD (University of Virginia), Douglas Gentile, PhD (Iowa State University), Faye Jones, MD (University of Louisville), James Perrin, MD, and Michael Jellinek, MD (Harvard University), and Thomas Boyle, PhD (University of

California at San Francisco). Many University of Rochester faculty members were also presenters at these Grand Rounds, including Drs. Mruzek, Iadarola, Silverman, and Smith.

Dr. Friedman died in 2013 (Sharkey, 2013). A conference in his memory assembled his trainees and many of the colleagues who started with him in the 1960s at the University of Rochester. Dr. Hyman worked with the Board of the Haggerty Friedman Foundation that included Dr. Haggerty, members of the Haggerty and Friedman families, and colleagues in NDBP from other institutions to examine resident and fellow training and the progression to include biopsychosocial influences in developmental diagnosis and care. A conference in honor of Dr. Haggerty shortly before his death in 2018 also brought former colleagues and trainees back to Rochester, who themselves have become international leaders. At Dr. Haggerty's request, the University of Rochester Medical Center established the Haggerty-Friedman Professorship in Developmental/Behavioral Pediatric Research with the funds that were donated. He lived to see Dr. Tristram Smith appointed as the first chair holder. Dr. Smith was the Haggerty-Friedman professor of Developmental/Behavioral Pediatric Research until his untimely death in 2018.

A fourth factor was receipt of several important legacy endowments were created during this period. In 2014, Dr. and Mrs. Davidson and their family created a legacy endowment that, upon their deaths will fund a visiting scholar's program and at least one traineeship in IDD. The projects were named the Philip W. and Margaret B. Davidson Visiting Scholars Program and the Philip W. and Margaret B. Davidson Fellowship in IDD and were intended to complement the Haggerty-Friedman Project focused on Behavioral Pediatrics. Both the Visiting Professorship and the Fellowship are to be focused on research and research training in IDD. The Department of Pediatrics and NDBP decided to commence the Visiting Professorship. Stephen Schroeder, PhD, was the first Davidson scholar in 2016. He was followed by Dr. Sulkes in 2017, Drs. Smith and Foxe in 2018, Dr. Georgina Peacock from the Centers for Disease Control and Prevention in 2019, and Dr. Christy Petrenko and Ms. Cole in 2020. The 2021 lecture will be given by Dr. Hyman.

The Maudie Weeks Fund was established in 2005 with a gift from the Edwin R. Weeks and Maudie Weeks Trusts. Named in honor of their son "Eddie" who has Down syndrome, the purpose of the endowment is to support training of health care providers in the Finger Lakes Region and beyond, specifically related to the needs of adults with Down Syndrome and other developmental disability conditions. Oversight of the use of funds from the endowment is provided by Dr. John Ghertner, physician to Eddie upon his return to the Newark, New York, community after discharge from the Newark Developmental Center. The endowment has supported activities to train medical students, residents, and physicians in practice in care of people with IDD. It has supported training of physician and nursing specialists in family medicine, internal medicine, geriatrics, psychiatry, and rehabilitation medicine, as well as dentists and other providers. It has facilitated the development of medical school and residency curricula, and numerous continuing-education programs. It also has supported the UCEDD's work at the national level to reduce disparities in health and health access for people with IDD across their lifespans, including collaboration with Special Olympics and the American Academy of Developmental Medicine and Dentistry (AADMD). With the help of this fund, the University of Rochester became the home of the first AADMD student chapter to jointly include trainees in medicine, dentistry, and nursing.

Kerry and Paulette Kyle, Rochester citizens with an interest in developmental disabilities, began providing support for divisional projects in 2015. Their initial donation supported development of an Adolescent Lounge within the division's new clinical space at 200 East River Road. In 2016, the Kyle family supported the expansion of support for fellowship research activities, and for the development of a Developmental Disabilities Family Experience for residents in Pediatrics, Internal Medicine/Pediatrics, Family Medicine, Dentistry, and other subspecialties. This support allowed further expansion so that all Rochester third-year medical students now have a Family Experience.

Other significant endowments were established by the Skirboll Family (which established an annual conference on ASD), Dr. and Mrs. Winston Gaum, Joan Ryan, Jean and John Warren, and the Francis Family. The Corning Company endowed a program providing for family navigation for children and youth with developmental disabilities from the three-county region of the Southern Tier where their employees reside in addition to piloting telehealth.

A fifth major factor that influenced divisional culture as noted above was formal approval by the Accreditation Council for Graduate Medical Education (ACGME) of fellowship training in Development and Behavioral Pediatrics. Dr. Sulkes and all other pediatricians working in NDBP successfully completed Board certification and the NDBP pediatric fellowship was approved for ACGME certification. This also impacted the LEND curriculum for pediatric fellows and by extension other health-related professions participating in LEND training activities. The subspecialty fellowship in pediatrics in the division was in Developmental-Behavioral Pediatrics and the maturation of that recently Boarded subspecialty allowed for recognition by other pediatric divisions at the Golisano Children's Hospital. That clinical space allowed for colocation of DBP, Child Neurology and Child and Adolescent Psychiatry in one location to better serve the patients and to promote interprofessional training.

The name of the division was changed to Developmental and Behavioral Pediatrics (DBP) prior to the move of the clinical service to the new clinical building on East River Road in 2017. The name change paralleled the specialty board and distinguished the services from Child Neurology.

# Chapter Eleven

# BEYOND DREAMS

*Every great dream begins with a dreamer. Always remember, you have within you the strength, the patience, and the passion to reach for the stars to change the world.*

—Harriet Tubman

One of the first things that happened when the UCEDD became an entity within DBP was to clearly develop DBP's pediatric mission while enabling the UCEDD to continue its age-span focus required by its federal funding mandate. This task required innovation, in part because the UCEDD and the LEND training programs were closely aligned and much of DBP's interdisciplinary educational mission was funded through LEND. Hence LEND also began to change.

Several events promoted this change. First, construction began on the new Golisano Children's Hospital, which opened May 27, 2015. Before the opening, there was an increasing demand on all pediatric divisions to expand clinical service. In the case of DBP, this pressure came largely from the emerging demand for diagnostic and intervention services on behalf of children with ASD and their families. The historic UCEDD missions did not include clinical service, so the responsibility to expand services and supports fell to the divisional efforts of DBP. We will have more to say about DBP's clinical service expansion in Chapter Twelve.

Of immense importance related to DBP was B. Thomas Golisano's personal interest in IDD and his efforts to bring the Golisano Foundation and DBP closer together. Both the University of Rochester Medical Center leadership and the University of Rochester Advancement Office raised IDD to a level of prominence not seen before. And there was almost immediate impact.

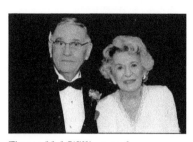

Figure 11.1 William and Mildred Levine. Photo from UR Advancement.

As plans were being finalized for the Golisano Children's Hospital construction, the University of Rochester Medical Center announced that a major gift from the William and Mildred Levine Foundation would be the impetus for a new building to house the URMC ASD Clinic. That building, located on East River Road, opened March 29, 2017. It houses the outpatient services of DBP, Child Neurology and Child and Adolescent Psychiatry as well as an imaging center, thus providing patients with the opportunity for integration of care and allowing for improved cross-disciplinary training on ASD and IDD.

A number of substantial gifts were made to support the Levine building. Two of these gifts were received from DBP faculty members. John and Kathy Purcell made a generous contribution to name the waiting area for families being seen at the ASD Clinic. And in early 2020 the Family Library was named to honor Susan L. Hyman following a gift from her family. Other gifts resulted in naming of the Teen Waiting Room (The Kyle Family), Child Life Room, Entrance lobby (Joan Ryan), and Sensory Room (Cornell/Weinstein Family).

A building on Science Parkway called the B. Thomas Golisano Institute for Behavioral Health, will offer day treatment and additional outpatient clinical space for the Division of Child and Adolescent Psychiatry. There is significant co-occurring behavioral health need among children and youth with ASD and their families. The Golisano Foundation has also funded a companion building on Science Parkway that will house both community organizations that provide family support around ASD and classrooms of existing school programs in the community, in addition to leisure and prevocational opportunities for individuals with ASD, called the Golisano Autism Center.

The Golisano Foundation also promoted the expansion of services and supports to address community health around the world through their connection with Special Olympics International (SoI). The Foundation and SoI worked together to create the Healthy Communities project, which seeks to improve fitness and health outcomes among athletes participating in SOI events and their families as well as the communities in which they live. This program includes sites in a number of locations including Rochester and has an age-span focus. Ann Costello, the Executive Director of the Golisano Foundation, turned to URMC to assume institutional leadership in this program and in turn involved DBP, including UCEDD-based faculty and staff. The impact of this collaboration was to further raise awareness of IDD at the highest level of the Medical Center Administration. Dr. Sulkes played a very large role in this process. In 2016 he received a Global Health Leadership award from SoI and in 2018, he was honored by the Golisano Foundation for his international work.

As the relationship between the Foundation and the Medical Center was unfolding, the UCEDD was advocating for the Department of Medicine to create a clinical option to assist older adolescents with IDD to transition to adult primary care medical services. In 2015 the Department of Medicine independently established the Complex Care Center to meet this need. This program is administratively managed through both the Department of Medicine and Pediatrics and is directed by Tiffany Pulcino, MD, MPH. Dr. Pulcino also leads the division of Transition Medicine in the Department of Pediatrics, which provides faculty support and programmatic guidance to transitioning youth with complex conditions, including IDD, to care by adult health providers. This primary care practice and inpatient presence accommodates adults with chronic illnesses with origins in childhood including ASD and IDD. The outpatient clinic is located near the Medicine-Pediatrics Resident practice on Culver Road. The clinic is designed to provide interdisciplinary care to adolescents and young adults with complex needs. It is staffed by residents and faculty in the Medicine-Pediatrics Residency Program with interdisciplinary care including dentistry, behavioral health, nursing, and nutrition. This clinic and its educational program address a long-standing need to improve expertise of providers needed to meet the primary health care needs of adults with IDD living in the community. As the clinic was emerging, DBP scaled down and eventually eliminated its focus on aging and IDD as other initiatives for children and youth became more focal. The UCEDD continued a focus on lifespan needs, including employment.

The collective influence on DBP of these events was dizzying, somewhat unexpected, and certainly not predictable. After over 50 years of development as a division within the Department of Pediatrics with little or no integration with strategic advancement with the Medical Center, DBP found itself included in the Medical Center Strategic Plan, at the center of construction planning, and most of all, in the midst of a very large expansion of clinical service.

In 2017 an IDD leadership Council was formed under the direction of Drs. Foxe and Pulcino to bring all IDD interests at URMC together for the benefit of the clinical research and advocacy missions. Dr. Pulcino, who is also the medical director of The URMC's Delivery System Reform Incentive Program (DISRP) assumed leadership of clinical primary care for adults with IDD. This leadership group now included DBP (Dr Hyman), LEND (Dr. Sulkes transitioning to Drs. Silverman and Kroening), SCDD (Dr. Hetherington transitioning to Dr. Iadarola), and leadership from the Eastman Dental School, Martha Mock, PhD, from the Warner School, Social Work, and the chairs of Pediatrics, Medicine, Psychiatry, and Neurology. A working group on Behavioral Health needs of persons with IDD includes represented faculty from the Complex Care Clinic (Dr. Pulcino), DBP (Drs. Hyman, McAdam, and Mruzek), Social Work (Lisa Luxemberg), Psychiatry (Dr. Michael Scharf), and URMC Board Member Anne Francis, MD.

An added benefit of AS ATN participation has been the increased involvement of families and self-advocates in clinical planning, research, and training. This training extends to families and community members. AS ATN funding supplemented by donations from Autism Up and private individuals provide for Family Navigation to help newly diagnosed families and families at life transitions access community resources and support. The Family Advisory Committee of the Rochester site of the AS ATN recommended that an annual conference for the community on research updates from Rochester and the AS ATN be staged. The first conference was in 2012. As mentioned earlier, the generous donation from the Skirboll Family has enhanced the possibilities for this conference since 2016 and allows it to be offered to the community annually as a means of providing evidence-based information that is useful to families.

# Chapter Twelve

# DBP'S CLINICAL PROGRAM EXPANDS

*. . . I am leading an effort [at URMC] to establish a culture in
which patients and families are an integral part of the health
care team. A culture in which patients feel safe asking questions
of their caregivers, where they experience the highest quality care.
A culture where providers have the courage to talk openly about
even the most difficult subjects. A culture that promotes compas-
sionate and attentive care for patients and for each other.*
—Bradford C. Berk, MD, PhD.

Clinical services at URMC began to change as early as the mid-1980s as managed care began to influence financing of health care. The driver for primary and subspecialty care in all disciplines shifted from providers to consumers. As health-care expenses continued to rise, insurers began to play an increasingly influential role in service design. By the year 2000, competition for covered lives intensified in Western New York, eventually creating three, and then two health systems, one managed by Strong Health and the other by Via Health. There was a re-alignment of primary care practices and referral networks with one or the other health system, and a dramatic expansion of community-based options for care. This shift is still occurring and has dictated the need for more primary care practices in the community and more clinical time from providers based in tertiary care centers such as Strong Memorial Hospital. Reimbursement for services was now based upon specific metrics such as Relative Value Units (RVUs); the more RVUs provided by a clinician, the more revenue generated from public and private insurance payers.

DBP had successfully negotiated with Blue Cross-Blue Shield several times during the 1980s and 1990s for comprehensive coverage for interdisciplinary services. It was now necessary to build similar comprehensiveness into the new reimbursement schemes. Third-party payers and health systems both recognized the need for such mechanisms in order to assure availability of clinical services to children and adults with ASD. Hence negotiations involving RVUs for comprehensive developmental services were now championed by administrative units within the Medical Center. So now there existed a perfect storm of sorts: demand from families for service and better mechanisms for reimbursement. Much of DBP's service expansion, even with better reimbursement, has been funded at least in part from state and local grants. However, with Medicaid waiver programs for youth with IDD, more and more patients served by DBP are insured through Medicaid with lower reimbursement for services provided than private insurers.

Figure 12.1 depicts the growth of clinical services, expressed in terms of the number of patients served per year, from 1986 to 2018: Dramatic growth indeed.

Beginning in 2012, DBP reorganized its existing clinical service programs under the leadership of Lynn Cole. People referred for any IDD diagnosis are first evaluated in a DBP Comprehensive Diagnostic Clinic, then either served by one or more treatment or consultation services or referred to a community resource.

## DBP Clinic

Children and youth with an array of developmental disorders including IDD, ASD, Down syndrome, developmental delays, and other complex developmental disorders are evaluated by clinicians for diagnosis in the DBP outpatient clinic. Data on cognitive, language, and adaptive function may be collected from school or early intervention settings for cost containment. Follow-up medical monitoring and developmental management is provided.

## Levine Autism Clinic

If a child is diagnosed with ASD, their continuing care takes place through the Levine Autism Clinic where faculty and staff have specialized knowledge in assessment and treatment planning for

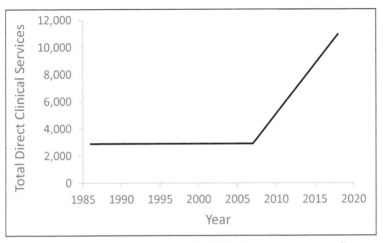

Figure 12.1. DBP Clinical Services 1986–2018. Data are consumer direct services for the years shown on the y-axis. Data for 1886 and 2007 were abstracted from the 1986 and 2007 DBP Annual Reports. Data for 2018 were summarized from the Department of Pediatrics database. Figure plotted by Don Harrington.

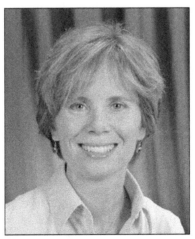

Figure 12.2. Lynn Cole, MSN, PNP. Reproduced with permission.

children and adolescents with ASD. Influenced by participation in the AS ATN, the clinical practice has reflected standardization of ASD diagnosis and follow-up care, inclusion of a family advisory committee, a Family Navigator program to provide support and guidance to both newly diagnosed families and those at life transitions, and participation in national Quality Improvement work through the Autism Health Learning Network.

## Infant and Toddler Development Program

As noted earlier, the NYSED stopped supporting its network of Early Childhood Direction Centers and DBP in turn closed the Neonatal Follow-up Program and replaced it with a Prenatal Consultation Service and an Infant-Toddler Developmental Program. Prenatal consultations were now provided for families who are carrying a fetus with a developmental disorder diagnosed during prenatal testing. Expectant parents are offered support and information about developmental disorders during the prenatal consultation. The Infant-Toddler program addresses the developmental needs of children born prematurely or who have health complications at birth. This has been extended to infants identified as having Neonatal Abstinence Syndrome (a group of complications following in-utero opiate exposure) in the newborn nursery. Prenatal exposure places these babies at high risk for developmental and behavioral problems.

## Physical Disabilities Program

The Andrew J. Kirch Developmental Services Center was renamed with a narrowed focus to providing multidisciplinary services to children and adolescents with motor development disorders. This program includes multidisciplinary care with child neurology (through a jointly appointed Neurodevelopmental Disabilities Boarded Child Neurology faculty member, Jennifer Nguyen, MD), Orthopedics, Nursing, Physical Therapy, Occupational Therapy and Social Work. The lead nurse practitioner for this program is Lorna Patanella, RN, PNP.

## FASD Clinic

In 2013, a Fetal Alcohol Spectrum Disorders (FASD) Clinic began. This clinic is a collaboration between DBP and the Mount Hope Family Center and provides diagnosis and intervention services for children in the Western and Central NY region in need of FASD diagnosis. It sees between 10 and 15 children per month. An increasing number of referrals are to evaluate children who experience significant psychosocial trauma and are at developmental and behavioral risk. It is led by Christie Petrenko, PhD, and Lynn Cole, PNP, with support from Abigail Kroening, MD, Lisa Luxemberg LCSW, and others.

## Behavioral Services

By far the largest increase in service took place in new behavioral services for children with ASD and their parents.

### Feeding Disorders Clinic

In 2012, DBP formalized a Pediatric Feeding Disorders Program, now staffed by two psychologists (Kimberly Brown, PhD, joined by Courtney Aponte, PhD, two nutritionists, and a speech/language pathologist. This program addresses feeding disorders found frequently in children with ASD and other developmental disabilities. Because of the need for evidence-based feeding interventions for young children with medical disorders, they will also see children referred by other divisions, such as allergy and gastroenterology.

### Behavioral Intervention for Families (BIFF)

In 2009, NDBP introduced Manualized Parent Training and Behavioral Intervention for Families program based on the dramatic results of the RUBI study (described in Chapter 13) examining parent mediated interventions. This rapid implementation in a clinical setting of an evidence-based intervention tested in a URMC research study demonstrates the integration of research and clinical care in DBP. The BIFF program was developed by Laura Silverman, PhD.

## Behavior Treatment Program

In 2014, the Behavior Treatment Program was initiated with funding from the Greater Rochester Health Foundation to address the unmet behavioral needs of children and youth with ASD. Using an evidence-based approach of applied behavior analysis, families became participants in effecting behavior change for targeted more severe behaviors, like tantrums, aggression, and self-injurious behavior. This is designed as a time-limited and focused intervention to manage access for the large number of families in need. It was initially developed by Carolyn Magyar, PhD. It is now led by Kenneth Shamlian, PsyD.

## Crisis Intervention

The long-standing crisis intervention program funded by NYS OPWDD receives most of its referrals from the clinical services of DBP (described previously).

## Corning Collaboration

In 2018, DBP received a grant from the Corning Health Services to enhance services and coordination of care for families in the Southern Tier. This project, led by Lynn Cole, PNP, includes dedicated support to start and test a Telemedicine Program. This project made it possible for families in the Southern Tier to receive virtual medical follow-up and behavioral therapy from DBP without having to travel to Rochester. DBP also undertook a leadership role in coordinating information and referral services to exiting services and supports based in the Southern Tier, while maintaining links to each service on the DBP website.

## Community Consultation Program (CCP)

Between 2008 and 2018, the Community Consultation Program Team increased its outreach services to individuals, agencies, and schools located throughout the Finger Lakes Region, sometimes located as far away as a two-hour drive to Rochester. CCP has continued to evolve. As school districts have hired their own behavior specialists, the faculty in CCP have increasingly provided programmatic consultation and joined the faculty of the Warner School to train Board Certified Behavior Analysts to serve the region.

A larger number of clinical hours to deliver the new or expanded services required increasing clinical time of existing DBP faculty and staff as well as adding newly recruited personnel. Many faculty and staff have activities in multiple areas which marry their clinical, research, teaching, and administrative duties. This has resulted in greater interaction between functional areas and with communication with community partners. It also recognizes the increasing importance of families and self-advocates as partners in the research process.

In 2017, the Rochester Business Journal recognized DBP as Disability Care Providers of the Year. A long journey from 1947!

# Chapter Thirteen

# DRAMATIC GROWTH OF
# AUTISM RESEARCH

*Start by doing what's necessary; then do what's possible; and
suddenly you are doing the impossible.*
—Francis of Assisi

Continuous funding from multiple sources for multiple projects is the key ingredient of programmatic research. Building on the research programs we discussed earlier, DBP was able to accomplish the incredible feat of maintaining and expanding the Seychelles Child Development Study while securing and retaining funding for programmatic research in ASD. Figure 13.1 shows the impact in US dollars of this growth. The most impressive growth took place in ASD research and the history is remarkable.

Treatment and intervention research were the focus of the efforts of the STAART Project and its participation in the AS ATN. The ASD research group expanded both group and single case study design research, with recruitment of participants from the DBP clinical services, from the ATN, and from the division's numerous community connections. Larger numbers permitted larger group designs and more specific studies (Hyman et al., 2016).

In 2008, Dr. Smith recruited Laura Silverman, PhD. Dr. Silverman joined the division after completion of her postdoctoral fellowship. In addition to clinical responsibilities, she built on the work in gesture and communication started in her doctoral work with Dr. Bennetto. She pursued additional translational studies with Lisbeth Romanski, PhD, using the same paradigms to study gesture understanding in humans and primates.

A second portentous faculty recruit was Suzannah Iadarola, PhD. Dr. Iadarola had been a research assistant in the STAART

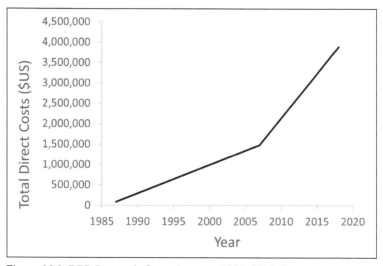

Figure 13.1. DBP Research Grant Income, 1986–2018, Data are
expressed in total direct costs. Data for 1986 and 2007 are from DBP
Annual Reports for those years. Data for 2018 were obtained from the
Department of Pediatrics. Figure plotted by Don Harrington.

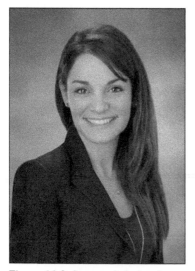

Figure 13.2. Susannah Iadorola,
PhD. Photo from Dr. Iadorola
and reproduced with permission.

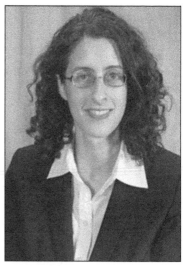

Figure 13.3. Laura Silverman,
PhD. Reproduced with
permission.

program prior to obtaining her PhD with Sandra Harris, PhD, at Rutgers University and completing a pre- and postdoctoral fellowship at Children's Hospital of Philadelphia. Dr. Iadarola was mentored by Dr. Smith and collaborated with him in the promotion of the understanding of the interface of behavioral and developmental approaches to intervention. Her very exciting NIH Research Scientist Development Award investigated the stress experienced by families of children with autism and how that impacted intervention.

## The Smith Legacy

With collaborators across the division, Dr. Smith led the University of Rochester to prominence in funded intervention research related to ASD. In his years at Rochester, Dr. Smith extended his seminal work establishing Early Intensive Behavioral Intervention as an evidence-based intervention to confirming the efficacy in community application and extending the evidence base to family participation in behavioral intervention.

### CHARTS (Children with Hyperactivity and Autism Research Treatment Study)

Dr. Smith established collaboration with Michael Aman, PhD, of the Nisonger Center at the Ohio State University and one of the world's leading experts on psychopharmacology and IDD (Aman et al., 2018). DBP joined the CHARTS network based at the Ohio State University and including the University of Rochester and the University of Pittsburgh. This network undertook multicenter clinical trials of behavioral interventions and medication (Silverman et al., 2014). Specifically, the CHARTS group evaluated the comparative effects of atomoxetine, parent training, and their combination on ADHD symptoms in children with ASD (Handen et al., 2015). Collaborators in this work included Drs. Silverman and Hyman and NPs Melissa Ryan and Patricia Corbett-Dick.

## RUBI (Research Units on Behavioral Intervention)

To extend applications of parent training interventions, another collaboration was established with Larry Scahill, PhD, then of Yale University (now of Emory University) and enabling DBP to join Dr. Scahill's RUBI study. This project was designed as a multicenter clinical trial comparing parent training to psychoeducation on the disruptive behavior and noncompliance in children with ASD (Bearss et al., 2015), as well as parental stress (Iadarola et al., 2018a). Collaborators in this work included Drs. Iadarola, Silverman, and Oakes.

## Autism Center of Excellence (ACE)

During this same period, Dr. Smith extended his collaboration with Connie Kasari, PhD, at UCLA's Center for Autism Research and Treatment (CART) to participate in their Autism Center of Excellence (ACE) consortium. The ACE Program was established by the National Institutes of Health (NIH) to support large research projects on ASD. Only a few such grants have been funded. Enough funds are provided to support multicenter large-scale studies directed at answering the same question. This collaboration enabled the Kasari and Smith team to evaluate the relative efficacy of more adult-directed discrete trial teaching approaches to more child-directed, social-communication focused intervention, specifically for increasing language in school-aged children with ASD with minimal vocal language. An additional extension of this work was that therapy was delivered in natural settings and included a parent training component. Other faculty who participated on this project included Drs. Iadarola and Levato.

## AIR-B (Autism Intervention Research–Behavioral)

Dr. Smith's research continued to gather momentum. In collaboration with Dr. Kasari, DBP became a site for an Autism Intervention Research Network on Behavioral Health (AIR-B). The focus of this is to address the well-documented race, ethnicity, and income-based disparities in ASD. The AIR-B network includes UCLA, The University of Pennsylvania, University of California at

Davis, Drexel University, and the University of Rochester. This network has conducted several randomized controlled trials (RCT) in underserved schools and communities. In DBP's first five-year cycle with AIR-B, interventions focused on reaching students with ASD in public schools. One RCT included a behavioral intervention to support transitions within the daily routine (Iadarola et al., 2018b). A second focused on teacher-mediated interventions to increase social engagement among students (including those with ASD) in inclusion settings (Shih et al., 2019). Currently, DBP is participating in a second cycle with AIR-B, running two concurrent RCTS: one to provide parent support and engagement following an ASD diagnosis and the other to support students with ASD transitioning into kindergarten, middle, or high school. Dr. Iadarola took over as PI in 2018 to carry on Dr. Smith's work.

### SAAGE (Students with Autism Accessing General Education)

Dr. Smith collaborated with Rose Iovannone, PhD, at the University of South Florida and Cynthia Anderson, PhD, at the May Institute, two established investigators conducting school-based intervention research, to implement SAAGE). SAAGE was a comprehensive, modular intervention for supporting students with ASD in classroom settings (Anderson et al., 2018; Lopata et al., 2018). This work was based on a clinically informed manual that was a collaborative work by the behaviorally oriented faculty who staffed the community consultation service through the division. Collaborators in the book that was the springboard for this project included Drs. Magyar, McAdam, Mruzek, Napolitano, and Linda Matons, EdM.

## Continuing the Smith Legacy

Dr. Smith was the Director of Research in DBP. This responsibility was given on an interim basis to Drs. Silverman and Iadarola after his death. At that time, the SAAGE, STAART, and AIR-B projects were transitioned to Dr. Iadarola's leadership. Dr. Smith had been preparing her for this role during the last year of his life when he took a well-deserved half-time sabbatical to prepare for the next chapter of his own research career: neurophysiologically informed or measured behavioral interventions. He had many other projects that were visionary, such as using natural language documentation to identify patients with ASD (Yuan et al., 2017). Without doubt, Dr. Smith's name and work will endure so long as there is at least one child with ASD on earth. It is now universally accepted that ABA can be delivered effectively by parents, caregivers, teachers, and other community-based providers, and that it has enduring fidelity (Waters et al., 2018). Dr. Smith gets most of the credit for those truths. At the time of his death, the warm words from his colleague Amanda Gulsrud included below were shared with the autism community:

> Tris had the best smile. That smile embodied the man he was—open, warm, and kind; qualities that are particularly remarkable for a person whose profession is measured by individual accomplishments. Yet Tris managed to be both extremely prolific in our field and also a team player among us, building up those around him with thoughtful encouragement and a listening ear. I was fortunate to have benefited from many years of friendship, mentorship and collegiality with Tris. Our AIR-B team and the world of autism research and treatment have suffered a great loss, but I am confident that his legacy will live on in the important work he accomplished and personal imprints he left with colleagues, friends, and families of individuals with ASD.
> —Dr. Amanda Gulsrud, UCLA, 2018.

## Additional Divisional Research on Interventions for ASD

Dr. Smith, as Research Director, supported other divisional faculty in their research applications and served as a mentor and coinvestigator on many projects examining interventions for ASD. These included the following:

### Toilet Training

Dr. Mruzek was funded through the Autism Treatment Network initially for a pilot project establishing the efficacy of a wireless moisture alarm in conjunction with a behavioral plan to teach toilet training to children with autism. This was subsequently funded to a multisite trial and to a school-based trial (Mruzek et al., 2019; Smith et al., 2014).

## Wandering and Elopement

Dr. McAdam was awarded funding by Autism Speaks to determine the factors that lead to elopement among children with ASD and plan behavioral interventions for this serious problem.

## Health Literacy for Youth with ASD

URMC faculty members (Drs. Smith, Silverman, Hetherington, Therese Welch, and Hyman) and Julie Christianson, PhD, at the University of Iowa used qualitative methods to evaluate the transition health needs of older adolescents with ASD and their parents in Rochester and develop and test a manualized intervention to improve health literacy. Overall leadership of this project was provided by Laura Shone, PhD, formally of URMC and now at the American Academy of Pediatrics.

## Translational Studies Examining Communication and Processing in ASD

NIH funding to Dr. Silverman allowed her to recruit and evaluate gesture communication and music perception in a cohort of teens with ASD compared to controls (Silverman et al., 2010). This work fit nicely with ongoing studies in Dr. Bennetto's lab on the River Campus that also were pursuing understanding of auditory processing.

## Bilirubin and ASD

Dr. Smith collaborated with Sanjiv Amin, MD, of the Division of Neonatology to investigate the potential role of hyperbilirubinemia on auditory processing and the potential association with ASD (Aman et al., 2019).

## AS ATN Registry

AS ATN funding required participation in the AS ATN registry that collected clinical data on consented participants in the first years of the registry. This data on over 7,000 children with ASD across AS ATN sites informed important advances in understanding the physical and behavioral health of participants ( Ameis et al., 2013; Bellesheim et al., 2018; Coury et al., 2012; deVinck-Baroody et al., 2015; Perrin et al., 2012). In the second cycle of funding, 50 of the over 400 children recruited in Rochester were re-evaluated to inform the first longitudinal data on health and behavioral health in youth with ASD. The AS ATN has moved from demographic description to the use of Quality Improvement methodology to impact patient care. The third cycle of AS ATN funding resulted in additional support from HRSA through the Autism Intervention Research–Physical (AIR-P) program at Massachusetts General Hospital. DBP is participating in the Autism Health Learning Network Database (AHLN), which is focused on harnessing the power of the EMR, parent reported outcome measures and change management to improve care in the clinical settings at the AS ATN sites and more widely through dissemination efforts.

## AS ATN Diet and Nutrition Study

The first signature study funded by AS ATN was a multisite investigation of the nutrition of children with ASD across five ATN sites (University of Arkansas: Jill James, PhD; University of Cincinnati: Patricia Manning, MD; University of Colorado: Anne Reynolds, MD; and the University of Pittsburgh: Cynthia Johnson, PhD). Dr. Hyman provided overall leadership in collaboration with Patricia Stewart, PhD, and Brianne Schmidt, RD, in Rochester. This study documented with careful methodology that children with ASD had similar nutritional deficits to other children in America but were at additional risk for specific nutritional deficits (Hyman et al., 2012; Johnson et al., 2014; Johnson et al., 2019; Reynolds et al., 2012; Stewart et al., 2015).

## Sleep, Iron Deficiency, and ASD

Rochester was a site for a pilot project examining the association of decreased iron stores and sleep problems in children with ASD. The Rochester site was led by AS ATN collaborator Heidi Connolly, MD, of Sleep Medicine, with Drs. Hyman and Reiffer as collaborators (Malow et al., 2016).

## Influences of the AS ATN on Clinical Practice

The quality improvement methodology used to examine diagnostic and management practices through the AS ATN impacted the overall approach to care in the clinical setting. Ms. Cole became an expert in the use of Quality Improvement in clinical practice change with national leadership in the AS ATN Executive Committee. This quality improvement effort includes faculty and staff in addressing projects to enhance diagnosis and care. The site Quality Improvement lead is Brenna Cavanaugh, PsyD, since 2019, with mentorship by Ms. Cole.

DBP takes great pride in carrying out Dr. Smith's legacy and leading a multisite effort to compare Early Intense Behavioral Intervention with a modular applied behavior analysis approach funded by the Department of Defense funded in 2018. Dr. Hyman is site project leader with collaborators Drs. Iadarola and Levato. This is being carried out as envisioned by Dr. Smith with collaborators at Cleveland Clinic (Cynthia Johnson, PhD), May Institute (Cynthia Anderson, PhD), Vanderbilt University (Zachary Warren, PhD), and Nationwide Children's Hospital (Eric Butter, PhD). Over the past decade there have been many collaborations formed across the university to integrate basic and behavioral approaches to research.

# Trainee Research

With ACGME accreditation of the Developmental Behavioral Pediatrics Fellowship in 2008, fellows were expected to complete a meaningful research project with faculty supervision. DBP fellow Jessica Roesser (Reiffer), MD, published a study looking at genetic

diagnostics in autism; Kimberly Johnson, MD, examined gastroin-
testinal symptoms of children with autism; and DBP Fellows Jara
Johnson, DO, and Robert Nutt, MD, both completed projects as
part of the MPH degree requirements. Dr. Johnson studied the
seasonality of births of children with ASD given hypotheses about
maternal influenza exposure as etiologic, and Dr. Nutt studied
the qualitative experience of families whose new-borns did not
pass their hearing screening. Abigail Kroening, MD, studied the
cultural experience related to developmental delay in refugee
populations, Stephanie Straka, DO, studied the risk factors for
obesity in youth with ASD, and Jenniffer Herrera, MD, studied
ethnic disparity in diagnosis of Hispanic children in Rochester.
Emily Knight, MD, PhD, is studying auditory processing in youth
with ASD compared to controls in the laboratory of John Foxe,
PhD. All completed projects were presented at national meetings,
including the Pediatric Academic Societies, International Society
for Autism Research, and Society for Developmental and Behavioral Pediatrics. Postdoctoral fellows in psychology participated
in funded research projects to advance their skills and prepare
them for faculty positions. Undergraduate research assistants
have played an important role in completing funded studies and
have sought out research experiences related to ASD (Sham &
Smith, 2014). In addition, trainees in the LEND program also are
exposed to research; some of their research projects have resulted
in meaningful publications (Liptak et al., 2008).

# Chapter Fourteen

# CHANGING RELATIONSHIPS

*This act is powerful in its simplicity. It will ensure that people
with disabilities are given the basic guarantees for which they
have worked so long and so hard: independence, freedom of
choice, control of their lives, the opportunity to blend fully and
equally into the rich mosaic of the American mainstream.*

—President George H. W. Bush, remarks at the signing of
the Americans with Disabilities Act, July 26, 1990

The UCEDD and LEND are now integrated within the DBP as
an academic, educational and research entity. To fulfill both
URMC and community expectations the combined programs
developed complimentary foci and continued the integrated programmatic structure that existed historically.

As DBP expanded its pediatric clinical and research programs,
SCDD, while still providing substantial infrastructure for DBP,
used its resources to develop a renewed community based, age-
span identity and focused on health disparities, employment and
the need for recreation for people with IDD. LEND developed
novel approaches as well as the continuing educational infrastructure for traditional trainees and community members.

In 2008, the Golisano Foundation funded the Institute for
Innovative Transition, shared between SCDD and the Warner
Graduate School of Education and Human Development. The
project began with a community task force led by The Advocacy
Center (a local not-for-profit agency) and the Golisano Foundation, which issued a report calling for programs to facilitate the
transition from school to adulthood for young adults with IDD.
The project was headed by Dr. Martha Mock and Dr. Hetherington
and was housed in SCDD. The aim was to improve the quality of
life for individuals with IDD and their families as they transition

from school age to adulthood. The project's principal components included information dissemination and technical assistance to families and young adults through an information and referral center, community technical assistance to support the development of transition programs and activities, including site evaluation of current programs; young adult leadership council and speakers bureau; and outreach and technical assistance to area schools, colleges, and universities to facilitate campus-based opportunities for students with IDD, and innovative education and job-training programs.

A cornerstone of the initiative was Project SEARCH, a one-year high school transition program that provides training and education leading to employment for individuals with significant disabilities; and a campus-based college experience, Transition and Postsecondary Programs for Students with Intellectual Disabilities. Project SEARCH is a nationwide program started in Cincinnati, Ohio over 20 years ago (Daston et al., 2012). Between 2008 and 2012, 12 Rochester Project SEARCH interns per year were selected from BOCES and Rochester City Schools and attended their last year of high school in a classroom based in a business while also doing three internships over the course of the year. One of the businesses was the University of Rochester Medical Center; the others were Wegmans Food Markets, Inc., and the City of Rochester. This program has been expanded to 20 sites throughout New York State with SCDD as the coordinator.

In 2012, Dr. Mock moved the Institute to the Warner School, and shifted its focus to transition to higher education. SCDD, however, expanded its role in Project SEARCH to include coordination of New York State SEARCH sites, and developed an employment initiative funded by the federal government. The employment initiative was a robust program addressing young adults in transition from school to work. It had the consequence of giving the UCEDD statewide and national presence. So significant was the shift towards adult programs that the URMC Dean's Office granted "Virtual Center" status to SCDD.

Every five years, UCEDDs are required to apply for competitive continuation funding. Each UCEDD must choose its priorities for the upcoming five-year period from a list of federal priorities.

Each UCEDD's Consumer Advisory Council plays a key role in setting these priorities. In 2014, SCDD's Community Advisory Council, which has grown to over 40 regularly attending members with a majority of family members and self-advocates, recommended that SCDD continue its focus on Employment, recognizing that the Governor's Office had modeled a statewide Employment First initiative on the UCEDD's work in that priority area. Three other additional priorities were also recommended, addressing health disparities, recreation and leisure, and education. The program development that ensued because of these additional priorities clearly defined the UCEDD as an age-span, community-focused center, operating from within DBP but with a unique identity. As evidence of this stature, SCDD was chosen to host a summit on disability, poverty, and employment in 2018. The summit was designed to serve as a stakeholders' meeting to develop and implement a plan of action to address the under- and unemployment of people with disabilities.

In 2018, SCDD was named as the Community Services Champion awarded by Catholic Charities Community Services of Rochester. The citation read as follows:

> Over the past 33 years, Strong Center of Developmental Disabilities' work has influenced policy changes and heightened awareness of the importance of community inclusion for individuals with developmental disabilities. In addition to serving as a "best practices" resource to agencies and educators, and resource for parents and families, the Center has also raised important advocacy issues of health disparities and under employment of individuals, sparking community conversations and programs like Project SEARCH to help make gains in these areas. The Center is an important partner and resource to our community and agency as we work to further our mission of inclusion, independence and individuality.

The intensification of focus of SCDD on consumer and family issues and participation of consumers in governance of the UCEDD were mirrored in its education efforts. In 2008, the LEND program added an Advocacy discipline, coordinated by Jackie Yingling, followed by Carrie Burkin. In 2014, the discipline was expanded to include self-advocacy, coordinated by Jeiri Flores. In

2017, faculty from the division began offering a 10-week medical humanities seminar for second-year medical students.

At the end of 2018, DBP had accomplished goals that those of us who worked in the program at its beginning could only imagine. But it took over 60 years and we are not there yet!

# EPILOGUE

*The best way to predict the future is to create it.*
—Abraham Lincoln

The Merriam-Webster dictionary defines "epilogue" as a concluding section that rounds out the design of a literary work. Not included in this definition is the motivation for writing the book. Why was the book written? Why should anyone care if the book was ever written? How important is this story for the future leaders and implementers of IDD programs at the University of Rochester? Are there lessons in the narrative that can guide program developers in disciplines other than IDD, or Pediatrics, or Medicine, or academia, for that matter?

This book tells the story of a journey that began with a one small clinic in one department staffed by one faculty member which served a limited number of consumers. Over the ensuing six decades, these humble roots spawned a well-funded, multifaceted effort employing 88 faculty and staff members, which now affects the lives of thousands of people. What are we to make of this remarkable growth? First, the journey is not over. In fact, we would argue that it has embodied a common theme of the need for human service punctuated by episodes of opportunity for change, good and bad luck, unanticipated serendipity, and timing. Most of all, it has a base of principled and well-intentioned leadership, rooted in sound philosophy and genuine concern for the needs of people with IDD and their families. These human needs are not going to go away any time soon; thus, continued program development is bound to occur. But principled and well-intentioned leadership could easily be disrupted, ultimately undermining the program's future trajectory and even its survival.

Successful change in any setting, but particularly in academia, requires development and maintenance of partnerships. Almost every new initiative in our history has involved partnering with individuals or groups outside the DBP organization. Future

growth will depend even more on these and other, newer partnerships. There are already such forces at work. For example, the
development of an integrated and focused approach to basic science within the Neuroscience Institute and application for IDDRC
funding. This brings with it many opportunities. The focus on
translational science places a spotlight on basic science. In other
words, an integrated IDD Research Center may be the first step in
a URMC-wide expansion of focus on IDD. This will require a collaborative leadership system that will involve extant IDD programs,
including the programs of DBP and the UCEDD, as part of a larger
whole. The funding of the Rochester IDDRC presents an enor-
mous opportunity to build on existing strengths and the history
of clinical, clinical research, education, and community programs
related to IDD at UR. But it will take very careful planning. Of
course, this outcome would be very good news for IDD consumers
in Rochester and is consistent with the vision that guided program
development in the 1970s. At the same time, it must reflect the
history of DBP and the UCEDD responding to the service needs of
the community and the extant clinical, clinical research, training,
and advocacy infrastructure and activities.

Another example of an important partnership for DBP is its
relationship with the Department of Medicine's Complex Care
Center. Ever since the beginning of the UCEDD, its leadership
had been seeking a closer tie to the Department of Medicine.
There were several obvious reasons why this made sense. First, not
all people with IDD are children. In the mid-20th Century, pediatricians rendered health care and allied services to families with
children with IDD. Most offspring with IDD were placed in institutions when they reached maturity. As we have seen earlier in this
narrative, such arrangements were unacceptable to many families;
anyway, institutions were destined to become ugly relics of unfor-
tunate history. With more and more adults with IDD choosing to
reside in the community, there was going to be a need at some
stage for Internists, Medicine-Pediatrics, and Family Practice physicians to begin including people with IDD in their practices. To
accomplish this, more experience during medical education and
residency would be required.

Another need for partnering is the shifting demography
within the universe of people with IDD: More and more people

with IDD were surviving into adulthood and older age (Janicki et al., 1999). By the year 2000, over two thirds of people with IDD were adults and the fastest growth was occurring in the eighth decade of life. This trend has continued. The URMC and the IDD community alike were and probably are still not prepared for this shift in need. The Departments of Medicine, Family Medicine, Psychiatry, Neurology, and all the rest of the medical center's adult subspecialty departments are obvious partners to bring change. DBP may not be the only leader in this effort, as has been clear from the short recent history of the emergence of the Complex Care Center, but DBP has an important leadership role, as it has always filled, as the subspecialty within pediatrics that focuses on the causes, identification, and treatment of individuals with developmental disabilities and the divisional home of the LEND and UCEDD programs. The academic departments committed to care and research in IDD may be shifting; but the knowledge base, experience, and connections to the community historically lie with DBP. As this happens, we all need to remember Lincoln's advice.

DBP's foundation is cemented by an unwavering dedication to serving people with IDD and their families. It is also layered and laced with the parallel commitment to community partnerships to achieve excellence in programs and services outside the walls of the Medical center. These objectives are in DBP's DNA and must continue as its highest priority. To survive and thrive as an academic unit inside those walls, DBP must continue its pursuit of education and research at the highest level. Service, education, and research must also be intertwined, as they are now in DBP. This is a tall order. Successful researchers are not often weekend warriors. Health-care education depends very frequently upon supervised experience garnered in state-of-the-science clinical programs. Good teaching can take time away from service. The point here is that funding is fundamental to continued growth as a three-pronged center. DBP is lucky to have decades of continuous support for UCEDD and LEND administrative and core activities, which has served to keep the an active and involved cohort of faculty and staff firmly positioned between the Medical center and the community. It is important for DBP to build new clinical and research programs in this same mold. To accomplish this goal, DBP and the grant funded LEND and UCEDD programs will need to rely on their strong interdependent relationship, good leadership, good timing, and a bit of luck.

A focus on individuals with autism and other developmental disabilities are included in the medical center's strategic plan (something which few of us could have imagined ever happening). This position opens opportunities for seeking support through the University's Advancement Office. One focus is on ASD, given the rapid rise in prevalence and need for community resources. We cannot easily see far enough ahead to predict the needs of people with IDD and their families 20, 30, or 50 years from now. Building for the present, though, in some ways secures the future. For example, DBP provides evaluations and interventions for over 1,500 children and youth for ASD and other developmental disabilities each year. This group of consumers will be adults or older adults in 30 years. On the way, they all require evidence-based and effective interventions in early childhood, innovative postsecondary education, adult residential options, gainful employment, and recreation options, some of which do not yet exist, and ultimately, older-age health care. The integrated programs of DBP, LEND, the UCEDD and now colleagues across UR have made a start in this arena; but much more needs to be done.

What of other intellectual, developmental, and behavioral challenges that have not yet reached our level of awareness? Almost all DBP's accomplishments have occurred in reaction to existing or emerging community threats to people with IDD and their families. Can we see any on the horizon that might be proactively addressed? How about the potential re-emergence of eugenics as a result of the rapidly developing field of gene editing? At this stage, ethicists are worrying about this issue (Reinders et al., 2020). What about the potential spread of infectious diseases such as measles that is already occurring in undervaccinated areas around the world, including the United States (Hussain et al., 2018)? Further, we are finishing this book amid the Covid-19 pandemic, which had so far killed more than five hundred thousand US citizens. There is a role for experts in IDD to work with acute-care providers in the management of patients with disabilities who may be at higher risk for infection and complications, as well as with public health experts in behavioral interventions to teach masking and other preventive measures. These and other projects looking into the future take time, and people are busy. But recall Santayana's (1905) admonition about remembering the past.

This story is about sustained growth leading to change. Growth that promotes and guides change is underpinned by inspiration, innovation, effects on the human condition, and personal and professional commitment.

And that (together with some love) is why we wrote this book. *Meliora!*

# ACKNOWLEDGMENTS

Costs for publishing this book were provided by the Division of Developmental and Behavioral Pediatrics' Strong Center for Developmental Disabilities (UCEDD), The Department of Pediatrics and Golisano Children's Hospital, the Division of Child Neurology of the Department of Neurology, the Ernest J. Del Monte Institute for Neuroscience and its new Intellectual and Developmental Disabilities Research Center, and an anonymous donor. We are very grateful to all for their generosity.

Contributions to this history were made by many, but special recognition is reserved for Elizabeth R. McAnarney (our former boss) who contributed the foreword and supported the project in many ways. We are also indebted to Susan Hetherington, Stephen B. Sulkes, Neal A. McNabb, Robert J. Haggerty, Elizabeth R. McAnarney, Suzannah Iadarola, Karin Theurer-Kaufman, Ruth J. Messinger, Jenny C. Overeynder, Lynn Cole, Laura B. Silverman, Abigail Kroening, Nancy N. Cain, Linda Quijano, Mack Kennedy, and Gary J. Myers. Dr. Myers spent many hours both relating history and editing numerous versions of the manuscript. We send special thanks to Don Harrington for plotting Figures 12.1 and 13.1 and to Dr. Davidson's friend Jerry Griffin, who edited many of the images.

Between 1947 and 2019, the Department of Pediatrics has had eight chairs. We are indebted to the most recent seven, Drs. Bradford, Haggerty, Smith, Hoekelman, McAnarney, Schor, and Brophy, all of whom supported Developmental and Behavioral Pediatrics both financially and programmatically. Obviously, DBP/SCDD's growth required new space, expanded departmental administrative support, and departmental partnerships to achieve the best possible faculty recruitments. Gradually, more and more grants and contracts management support from the Department was required as the DBP extramural funding portfolio expanded. All of these supports were forthcoming when required with enthusiasm from departmental leadership. When DBP needed institutional buy-in for projects, each chairperson was there to smooth the way.

Many of the DBP programs we have written about were accomplished only because of collaboration with other divisions of the Department of Pediatrics. In our experience, these collaborations were productive in large part because they would result in services and supports for people with IDD and their families. But there were many other reasons, including the willingness and openness of interdivisional colleagues to partner with us. At Golisano Children's Hospital, it has always been about cooperative and collegial partnerships.

Literally hundreds of faculty members, fellows, and students worked in DBP programs. As any one of them would tell you, it was hard work. But without them, there would be no DBP story to be told.

We are in debt to Sonia Kane, editorial director of the University of Rochester Press, and Robert Kraus, chair of the press's editorial board, for their kind support and excellent suggestions throughout the past two years of the project, culminating in the final production of the book. It was a pleasure to work with them. Sue Smith, managing director editor of the press's publishing partner Boydell & Brewer Inc., was particularly helpful as well.

The first author has been supported for 54 years by his wife Margaret. She has done many things for him that may not have always been her first choice for how she spends her time. Editing the manuscript is surely one of those things. Her enthusiasm for the project grew with each page she cleaned up (PWD is not a particularly facile writer) and by the end of her "read," she said: "You two have done a good thing." We appreciate the compliment and hope she is right.

DBP began as a service to the community and service has remained a hallmark of its purpose for over 72 years. Thousands of consumers and their families have participating in DBP services and supports. The future will see many more thousands seek its help. We dedicated this book to one of them, Peg Sheehan. Peg is a friend of the first author. She also is a representative of the many thousands of people whose lives we hope were made better by DBP.

—PWD and SLH

# LIST OF ABBREVIATIONS

| | |
|---|---|
| AAB | Academic Advisory Board |
| AADMD | American Academy of Developmental Medicine and Dentistry |
| ACE | Autism Center of Excellence |
| ACGME | Accreditation Council for Graduate Medical Education |
| ADD | US Administration on Developmental Disabilities |
| ADHD | Attention Deficit Hyperactivity Disorder |
| AHLN | Autism Health Learning Network |
| AIR-B | Autism Intervention Research – Behavioral |
| AIR-P | Autism Intervention Research – Physical |
| AS-ATN | Autism Speaks–Autism Treatment Network |
| ASD | Autism Spectrum Disorder |
| AUCD | Association of University Centers on Disabilities |
| BDC | Birth Defects Center |
| BIFF | Behavioral Interventions for Families |
| BOCES | Board of Cooperative Educational Services |
| CAB | Community Advisory Board |
| CAC | Consumer Advisory Council |
| CART | UCLA's Center for Autism Research and Treatment |
| CCCIC | Coordination of Care for Chronically Ill Children |
| CCP | Community Consultation Program |
| CDC | Community Diagnostic Clinic |

| | |
|---|---|
| CHARTS | Children with Hyperactivity and Autism Research Treatment Study |
| CI | Crisis Intervention |
| C-MEDD | Consortium for Medical Education in Developmental Disabilities |
| CPEA | Collaborative Programs for Excellence in Autism |
| DBP | Developmental and Behavioral Pediatrics |
| DCDD | Diagnostic Clinic for Developmental Disabilities |
| DDO | US Developmental Disabilities Office |
| Developmental Center | New York State designation for congregate care institutions |
| DSRIP | University of Rochester Medical Center Delivery System Reform Incentive Program |
| EMR | Electronic Medical Record |
| FASD | Fetal Alcohol Spectrum Disorders |
| FLCDC | Finger Lakes Convulsive Disorders Center |
| FLDDSO | Finger Lakes Developmental Disabilities Services Office |
| HSRA | US Health Resources and Services Administration |
| IDD | Intellectual and Developmental Disabilities |
| IDDRC | Intellectual and Developmental Disabilities Research Center |
| IDEA | Individuals with Disabilities Education Act |
| K Award | NIH Research Career Development Award |
| LEND | Leadership Education in Neurodevelopmental and Related Disabilities |
| MCHB | US Maternal and Child Health Bureau |
| MDC | Monroe Developmental Center |
| MDU | Mobile Diagnostic Unit |

| | |
|---|---|
| MeHg | methylmercury |
| MRDD | Mental Retardation and Developmental Disabilities |
| MRDDRC | Mental Retardation and Developmental Disabilities Research Center |
| NCCP | Neonatal Continuing Care Program |
| NDBP | Neurodevelopmental and Behavioral Pediatrics |
| NICHD | Eunice Kennedy Shiver National Institute of Child Health and Human Development |
| NIH | National Institutes of Health |
| NYS | New York State |
| NYSDDPC | New York State Developmental Disabilities Planning Council |
| NYSED | New York State Education Department |
| OMRDD | New York State Office of Mental Retardation and Developmental Disabilities |
| OPWDD | New York State Office for People with Developmental Disabilities |
| PADD | Program on Aging and Developmental Disabilities |
| PoA | Partners of the Americas |
| PWD | Philip W. Davidson |
| RECDC | Regional Early Childhood Direction Center |
| RHSS | Rochester Health Status Survey |
| RUBI | Research Units on Behavioral Interventions |
| RVU | Relative Value Unit |
| SAAGE | Students with Autism Accessing General Education |
| SBS | Stephen Brian Sulkes |
| SCDD | Strong Center for Developmental Disabilities |
| SEARCH | Transition and Postsecondary Programs for Students with Intellectual Disabilities |

SLH            Susan L. Hyman

SoI            Special Olympics International

STAART         Studies to Advance Autism Research and Treatment

State School   Designation of New York State residential insti-
               tutions for people with intellectual and devel-
               opmental disabilities, which preceded the term
               *Development Center*

SUNY           State University of New York

TIP            Training Initiative Program

TPADD          Training Program on Aging and Developmental Dis-
               abilities

UADCDD         University Affiliated Diagnostic Clinic for Develop-
               mental Disorders

UAF            University Affiliated Facility

UAP            University Affiliated Program

UAPDD          University Affiliated Program on Developmental Dis-
               abilities

UCEDD          University Center of Excellence in Developmental
               Disabilities

UNC-CH         University of North Carolina at Chapel Hill

URMC           University of Rochester Medical Center

Willowbrook
Consent Decree Issued by Governor Wilson to direct the even-
               tual closure of New York State's Developmental
               Centers and transfer of residents to community-
               based programs

# REFERENCES

Aman, S. B., Smith. T., & Timler, G. (2019). Developmental influence of unconjugated hyperbilirubinemia and neurobehavioral disorders. *Pediatric Research*, *85*(2): 191–97. doi: 10.1038/s41390–018–0216–4. Epub 2018 Oct 23. Review.

Ameis, S. H., Corbett-Dick, P., Cole, L., & Correll, C. U. (2013). Decision making and antipsychotic medication treatment for youth with autism spectrum disorders: Applying guidelines in the real world. *Journal of Clinical Psychiatry*, *74*(10), 1022–4. doi: 10.4088/JCP.13ac08691.Amin-Zaki, L., Elhassani, S., Majeed, M. A., Clarkson. T. W., Doherty, R. A., & Greenwood, M. (1974). Intra-uterine methylmercury poisoning in Iraq. *Pediatrics*, *54*, 587–95.

Anderson, C. M., Smith. T., & Iovannone, R. (2018). Building capacity to support students with autism spectrum disorder: A Modular Approach to Intervention. *Education and Treatment of Children*, *41*(1): 107–37.

Bearss, K., Johnson. C., Smith, T., Lecavalier, L., Swiezy, N., Aman, M., & Sukhodolsky, D. G. (2015). Effect of parent training vs. parent education on behavioral problems in children with autism spectrum disorder: A randomized clinical trial. *Journal of the American Medical Association*, *313*(15): 1524–33.

Bellesheim, K. R., Cole, L., Coury, D. L., Yin, L., Levy, S. E., Guinnee, M. A., Klatka, K., Malow, B. A., Katz, T., Taylor, J., & Sohl, K. (2018). Family-driven goals to improve care for children with autism spectrum disorder. *Pediatrics*. *142*(3). pii: e20173225. doi: 10.1542/peds.2017–3225. Epub 2018 Aug 14.

Brown, J. A., Gram, M., & Kinnen, E. (1980). Parapodium design with knee and hip locks. *Orthotics and Prothesics*, *34*(2): 14–20.

*Children*, 1970, 17(6): 240.

Coury, D. L., Anagnostou, E., Manning-Courtney, P., Reynolds, A., Cole, L., McCoy, R., Whitaker, A., & Perrin, J. M. (2012). Use of psychotropic medication in children and adolescents with autism spectrum disorders. *Pediatrics, 130*, Suppl 2, S69–76. doi: 10.1542/peds.2012–0900D.

Daston, M., Reihle, E., & Rutkowski, S. (2012). *High School Transition That Works: Lessons Learned from Project SEARCH.* Paul Brookes Publishing.

Davidson, P. W., Reif, M., Shapiro, D., Griffith, B., Shapiro, P., & Crocker, A. C. (1984). Directional service: A model for secondary prevention of developmental handicapping conditions. *Mental Retardation, 22,* 21–27.

Davidson, P. W., & Fifield, M. G. (1985). The UAF satellite feasibility process: Experiences from 1984 and recommendations for the future. Report to the Commissioner, Administration on Developmental Disabilities. University of Rochester, New York (UAPDD printed report).

Davidson, P. W., Calkins, C., Burns, C. M., Sulkes, S. B., Chandler, C., & Bennett, F. (1986). Alternatives to federal support for funding of postgraduate clinical training and continuing education in developmental disabilities. *Applied Research in Mental Retardation, 8*(3): 487–98.

Davidson, P. W., Kendig, J., & Goode, D. (1992). University affiliated program sponsored consultation, technical assistance, and research in developing nations. *Mental Retardation, 30*(5): 269–76.

Davidson, P. W., Cain, N. N., Sloane-Reeves, J., Giesow, V., Quijano, L., VanHeyningen, J., & Shoham, I. (1995). Crisis intervention for community-based persons with developmental disabilities and concomitant behavioral and psychiatric disorders. *Mental Retardation, 33*(1): 21–30.

Davidson, P. W., Myers, G. J., Cox, C., Axtell, C., Shamlaye, C. F., Sloane-Reeves, J., Cernichiari, E., Choi, A., Wang, Y., Berlin, M., & Clarkson, T. W. (1998). Effects of prenatal and postnatal methylmercury exposure from fish consumption on neurodevelopment: Outcomes at 66 months of age in the Seychelles Child Development Study. *JAMA, 280*(8): 701–7.

Davidson, P. W., Morris, D., & Cain, N. N. (1999). Community services for persons with developmental disabilities and psychiatric or severe behavior disorders. In N. Bouras (Ed.), *Psychiatric and Behavioral Disorders in Developmental Disabilities and Mental Retardation.* Cambridge University Press, 359–72.

Davidson, P. W., Heller, T., Janicki, M. P., & Hyer, K. (2004). Defining a national research and practice agenda for older adults with intellectual disabilities. *Journal of Policy and Practice on Intellectual Disabilities, 1*(1): 2–9.

Davidson, P. W., Weiss, B., Beck, C., Cory-Slechta, D. A., Orlando, M., Loiselle, D., Young, E. C., Sloane-Reeves, J., & Myers, G. J. (2006). Development and validation of a test battery to assess subtle neurodevelopmental differences in children. *NeuroToxicology, 27,* 951–69.

Davidson, P. W., Strain, J. J., Myers, G. J., Thurston, S. W., Bonham, M. P., Shamlaye, C. F., Stokes-Riner, A., Wallace, J. M. W., Robson, P. J., Duffy, E. M., Georger, L. A., Sloane-Reeves, J., Cernichiari, E., Canfield, R. L., Cox. C., Huang, L-S., Janciuras, J., & Clarkson, T. W. (2008a). Neurodevelopmental effects of maternal nutritional status and exposure to methylmercury from eating fish during pregnancy. *NeuroToxicology, 29*(5): 767–75.

Davidson, P. W., Henderson, C. M., Janicki, M. P., Robinson, L. M., Bishop, K. M., Wells, A., Garroway. J., & Wexler, O. (2008b). Ascertaining health-related information on adults with intellectual disabilities: Development and field testing of the Rochester Health Status Survey. *Journal of Policy and Practice in Intellectual Disability,* 5(1), 12–23

de Vinck-Baroody, O., Shui, A., Macklin, E. A., Hyman, S. L., Leventhal, J. M., & Weitzman, C. (2015). Overweight and obesity in a sample of children with autism spectrum disorder. *Academic Pediatrics, 15*(4): 396–404. doi: 10.1016/j.acap.2015.03.008. Epub 2015 Apr 30.

Friedman, S. B. (1970). The challenge in behavioral pediatrics. *Journal of Pediatrics, 77*(1): 172–73.

Haggerty, R. J. (1968). Community pediatrics. *New England Journal of Medicine, 278,* 15– 21.

Haggerty, R. J. (1994). Community pediatrics: past and present. *Pediatric Annals, 23*(12): 657–58, 661–63.

Haggerty, R. J., & Friedman, S. B. (2003). History of developmental-behavioral pediatrics. Journal of Developmental and Behavioral Pediatrics, 24(1 Supplement): S1–18.

Haggerty, R. J., & Aligne, C. A. (2005). Community pediatrics: The Rochester story. Pediatrics, *115* (3 supplement).

Handen, B. L., Aman, M. G., Arnold, L. E., Hyman, S. L., Tumuluru, R. V., Lecavalier, L., & Silverman, L. B. (2015). Atomoxetine, parent training, and their combination in children with autism spectrum disorder and attention-deficit/hyperactivity disorder. *Journal of the American Academy of Child & Adolescent Psychiatry, 54*(11): 905–15.

Harada, Y. (1968). Congenital (or fetal) Minamata disease. In *Study Group of Minamata Disease* (pp. 93–117). Kumamoto University (Japan).

Henderson, C. M., & Davidson, P. W. (2000). Comprehensive adult and geriatric assessment. In M. P. Janicki & E. Ansello (Eds.), *Community supports for aging adults with lifelong disabilities* (pp. 373–86). Paul Brookes Publishing.

Hussain, A., Syed, A., Ahmed, M., & Hussain, S. (2018). The anti-vaccination movement: A regression in modern medicine. Cureus, 10(7), e2919.

Hyman, S. L., Stewart, P. A., Schmidt. B., Cain, U., Lemcke, N., Foley, J. T., Peck, R., Clemons, T., Reynolds, A., Johnson, C., Handen, B., James, S. J., Courtney, P. M., Molloy, C., & Ng, P. K. (2012). Nutrient intake from food in children with autism. *Pediatrics, 130*, Suppl 2, S145–53. doi: 10.1542/peds.2012–0900L.

Hyman, S. L., Stewart, P. A., Foley, J., Cain, U., Peck, R., Morris, D. D., Wang, H., & Smith, T. (2016). The gluten-free/casein-free diet: A double-blind challenge trial in children with autism. *Journal of Autism and Developmental Disorders. 46*(1): 205–20. doi: 10.1007/s10803–015–2564–9.

Iadarola, S., Levato, L., Harrison, B., Smith, T., Lecavalier, L., Johnson, C., & Scahill, L. (2018a). Teaching parents behavioral strategies for autism spectrum disorder (ASD): Effects on stress, strain, and competence. *Journal of Autism and Developmental Disorders, 48*(4): 1031–40.

Iadarola, S., Shih, W., Dean, M., Blanch, E., Harwood, R., Hetherington, S., & Smith T. (2018b). Implementing a manualized, classroom transition intervention for students with ASD in under-resourced schools. *Behavior Modification, 42*(1): 126–47.

Janicki, M. P., Dalton, A. R., Henderson, C. M., & Davidson, P. W. (1999). Mortality and morbidity among older adults with intellectual disabilities: Health services considerations. *Disability and Rehabilitation, 21*(5–6): 284–94.

Johnson, C. R., Turner, K., Stewart, P. A., Schmidt, B., Shui, A., Macklin, E., Reynolds, A., James, J., Johnson, S. L., Manning, C. P., & Hyman, S. L. (2014). Relationships between feeding problems, behavioral characteristics, and nutritional quality in children with ASD. *Journal of Autism and Developmental Disorders, 44*(9): 2175–84. doi: 10.1007/s10803-014-2095-9.

Johnson, C. R., Brown, K., Hyman, S. L., Brooks, M. M., Aponte, C., Levato, L., Schmidt, B., Evans, V., Huo, Z., Bendixen, R., Eng, H., Sax, T., & Smith, T. (2019). Parent training for feeding problems in children with autism spectrum disorder: Initial randomized trial. *Journal of Pediatric Psychology, 44*(2), 164–75.

Kaiser, J. (1996). Science Scope. *Science, 271*(5252), 1045.

Kroening, A. L., Moore, J. A., Welch, T. R., Halterman, J. S., & Hyman, S. L. (2016). Developmental screening of refugees: A qualitative study. Pediatrics, *138*(3). pii: e20160234. doi: 10.1542/peds.2016-0234. Epub 2016 Aug 15.

Larson, K. C. (2015). *Rosemary: The hidden Kennedy daughter.* Houghton Mifflin Harcourt.

Liptak, G. S., Burns, C. M., Davidson, P. W., & McAnarney, E. R. (1998). Effects of providing comprehensive ambulatory services to children with chronic conditions. *Archives of Pediatrics and Adolescent Medicine, 152,* 1003–8.

Liptak, G. S., Burns, C. M., McAnarney, E. R., & Davidson, P. W. (1999). Costs of care coordination for children with special health care needs. In reply. *Archives of Child and Adolescent Medicine, 153,* 1004.

Liptak, G. S., Benzoni, L. B., Mruzek, D. W., Nolan, K. W., Thingvoll, M. A., Wade, C. M., & Fryer, G. E. (2008). Disparities in diagnosis and access to health services for children with autism: Data from the National Survey of Children's Health. *Journal of Developmental and Behavioral Pediatrics, 29*(3): 152–60.

Llop, S., Tran, V., Ballester, F., Barbone, F., Sofianou-Katsoulis, A., Sunyer. J., Engström, K., Alhamdow, A., Love, T. M., Watson, G. E., Bustamante, M., Murcia, M., Shamlaye, C. F., Rosolen, V., Horvat, M., van Wijngaarden, E., Davidson, P. W., Myers, G. J., Rand, M. D., & Broberg, K. (2017). CYP3A genes and their association with prenatal methylmercury exposure and neurodevelopment. *Environment International, 105,* 34–42.

Lopata, C., Thomeer, M. L., Rodgers, J. D., Donnelly, J. P., McDonald, C. A., Volker, M. A., Smith, T. H., & Wang, H. (2018). Cluster randomized trial of a school intervention for children with autism spectrum disorder. *Journal of Clinical Child and Adolescent Psychology, 30*, 1–12. doi: 10.1080/15374416.2018.1520121. [Epub ahead of print]

Malow, B. A., Connolly, H. V., Weiss, S. K., Halbower, A., Goldman, S., Hyman, S. L., Katz, T., Madduri, N., Shui, A., Macklin, E., & Reynolds, A. M. (2016). The Pediatric Sleep Clinical Global Impressions Scale: A new tool to measure pediatric insomnia in autism spectrum disorders. *Journal of Developmental and Behavioral Pediatrics, 37*(5): 370–76. doi: 10.1097/DBP.0000000000000307.

Messinger, R., & Davidson, P. W. (1992). Training programs and defendants with mental retardation History and Future Direction. In R. W. Conley, R. Luckasson, & G. Bouthilet (Eds.), *The Criminal Justice System and Mental Retardation Defendants and Victims* (pp. 221–34). Paul H. Brookes.

Mruzek, D. W., McAleavey, S., Loring, W. A., Butter, E., Smith, T., McDonnell E., Levato, L., Aponte, C., Travis, R. P., Aiello, R. E., Taylor, C. M., Wilkins, J. W., Corbett-Dick, P., Finkelstein, D. M., York, A. M., & Zanibbi, K. (2019). A pilot investigation of an iOS-based app for toilet training children with autism spectrum disorder. *Autism. 23*(2): 359–70. doi: 10.1177/1362361317741741. Epub 2017 Dec 7.

Myers, G. J., Cerone, S. B., & Olson, A. L. (1981). *A guide for helping the child with spina bifida.* Charles C. Thomas.

Myers, G. J., Davidson, P. W., Cox, C., Huang, L-S., Palumbo, D., Cernichiari, E., Wilding, G., Sloane-Reeves, J., Kost, J., Shamlaye, C. F., & Clarkson, T. W. (2003). Prenatal methylmercury exposure from ocean fish consumption in the Seychelles Child Development Study. *The Lancet, 361*, 1686–92.

Nirje, B. (1969). The Normalization Principle and its human management implications. In R. B. Kugel & W. Wolfensberger (Eds.), *Changing patterns in residential services for the mentally retarded.* President's Committee on Mental Retardation, pp. 179–95.

Noll, S., & Trent, J. (Eds.) (2004) *Mental retardation in America: A historical reader.* New York University Press.

Pavlov, I. P. (1932). *Physiology of the higher nervous activity.* Moscow, Priroda, 93–94.

Perrin, J. M., Coury, D. L, Hyman, S. L., Cole, L., Reynolds, A. M., & Clemons, T. (2012). Complementary and alternative medicine use in a large pediatric autism sample. *Pediatrics, 130,* Suppl 2:S77–82. doi: 10.1542/peds.2012–0900E.

Pierson, S. S. (1893). The dedication. In *The New York State Custodial Asylum for Feeble-Minded Women Dedication Services* (pp. 8–28). P. D. Burgess.

President's Panel on Mental Retardation (1963). A National Plan to Combat Mental Retardation. (1963). *US Government Printing Office.*

Rafter, N. (2004). The criminalization of mental retardation. In S. Noll & J. W. Trent (Eds.), *Mental Retardation in America* (pp. 232–57). New York University Press.

Reinders, H. S., Stainton, T., & Parmenter, T. R. (2020). Disposable lives: Is ending the lives of persons with intellectual and developmental disabilities for reasons of poor quality of life an emergence of a new eugenics movement? In V. Prasher, P. W. Davidson, & F. H. Dos Santos (Eds.), *Mental health, intellectual and developmental disabilities, and the aging process (2nd ed.).* Springer Nature.

Reynolds, A., Krebs, N. F., Stewart, P. A., Austin, H., Johnson, S. L., Withrow, N., Molloy, C., James, S. J., Johnson, C., Clemons, T., Schmidt, B., & Hyman, S. L. (2012). Iron status in children with autism spectrum disorder. *Pediatrics, 130,* Suppl. 2, S154–9. doi: 10.1542/peds.2012–0900M.

Robert E. Cooke. Obituaries (2014). Legacy.com. https://www.legacy.com/obituaries/hartfordcourant/obituary.aspx?pid=169551094

Santayana, G. (1905). *The life of reason. Volume 1: Reason in common sense.* C. Scribner's & Sons.

Scheerenberger, R. C. (1987). *A history of mental retardation.* Paul H. Brookes.

Sham, E., & Smith, T. (2014). Publication bias in studies of an applied behavior-analytic intervention: An initial analysis. *Journal of Applied Behavior Analysis, 47*(3): 663–78. doi: 10.1002/jaba.146.

Sharkey, M. (2013). Stanford B. Friedman. MD *Journal of Developmental and Behavioral Pediatrics, 34*(6): 383.

Shih, W., Dean, M., Kretzmann, M., Locke, J., Senturk, D., Mandell, D. S., Kasari, C. (2019). Remaking recess intervention for improving peer interactions at school for children with autism spectrum disorder: multisite randomized trial. *School Psychology Review, 48*(2): 133–44.

Silverman, L. B., Bennetto, L., Campana, E., & Tanenhaus, M. K. (2010). Speech-and-gesture integration in high functioning autism.

*Cognition. 115*(3): 380–93. doi: 10.1016/j.cognition.2010.01.002. Epub 2010 Mar 30.

Silverman, L. B., Hollway, J. A., Smith, T., Aman, M. G., Arnold, L. E., Pan, X., & Handen, B. L. (2014). A multisite trial of atomoxetine and parent training in children with autism spectrum disorders: Rationale and design challenges. *Research in Autism Spectrum Disorders, 8*(7): 899–907.

Silverman, L. B., Eigsti, I. M., & Bennetto, L. (2017). I tawt i taw a puddy tat: Gestures in canary row narrations by high-functioning youth with autism spectrum disorder. *Autism Research, 10*(8), 1353–63. doi: 10.1002/aur.1785. Epub 2017 Apr 1.

Smith T. Field Report (2014, May 1).: Making toilet training easier: A novel enuresis alarm system. *Behavior Analytic Practice, 7*(1): 31–32. doi: 10.1007/s40617–014–0008–1. eCollection 2014 May.

*State of New York Board of Charities Report (1879).* Charles van Benthuysen & Sons. http://memory.loc.gov/service/gdc/scd0001/2010/20100727004an/20100727004an.pdf

Stearns, T. (2011). Early State Schools in New York. http://museumof disability.org/category/museum-of-disability-history-blog/

Stewart, P. A., Hyman, S. L., Schmidt, B. L., Macklin, E. A., Reynolds, A., Johnson. C. R., James, S. J., & Manning-Courtney, P. (2015). Dietary supplementation in children with autism spectrum disorders: Common, insufficient, and excessive. Journal of Academic Nutrition and Diet, *115*(8): 1237–48. doi: 10.1016/j. jand.2015.03.026.

Strain, J. J., Davidson, P. W., Bonham, M. P., Duffy, E. M., Stokes-Riner, A., Thurston, S. W., Wallace, J. M. W., Robson, P. J., Shamlaye, C. F., Georger, L. A., Sloane-Reeves, J., Cernichiari, E., Canfield, R. L., Cox. C., Huang, L-S., Janciuras, J., Myers, G. J., & Clarkson, T. W. (2008). Associations of maternal long chain polyunsaturated fatty acids, methylmercury, and infant development in the Seychelles Child Development and Nutrition Study. NeuroToxicology, 29(5): 776–82.

The Alan Mason Chesney Medical Archives of The Johns Hopkins Medical Institutions. The Robert E. Cooke Collection. *Johns Hopkins Medical Institutions.* https://medicalarchives.jhmi.edu:8443/papers/cooke.html

UCEDDs. *Association of University Centers of Excellence.* https://www.aucd.org/template/page.cfm?id=667.

University of Rochester Medical Center website. About David H. Smith, MD https://www.urmc.rochester.edu/cvbi/history.aspx

Vorojeikina, D., Broberg, K., Love, T. M., Davidson, P. W, vanWijngaarden, E., & Rand, M. D. (2017). Glutathione S-transferase activity moderates methylmercury toxicity during development in *drosophila. Toxicological Sciences, 157*(1): 211–21.

Waters, C. F., Amerine Dickens, M., Thurston, S. W., Lu, X., & Smith, T. (2018). Sustainability of early intensive behavioral intervention for children with autism spectrum disorder in a community setting. Behavior Modification, July 1: 145445518786463. doi: 10.1177/0145445518786463. [Epub ahead of print].

Watson, G. E., Lynch, M., Myers, G. J., Shamlaye, C. F., Thurston, S. W., Zareba, G., Clarkson, T. W., & Davidson, P. W. (2011). Prenatal exposure to dental amalgam: Reassuring evidence from the Seychelles Child Development main cohort, *Journal of the American Dental Association, 142*(11): 1283–94.

Watson, G. E., vanWijngaarden, E., Love, T., McSorley, E. M., Bonham, M. P., Mulhern, M. S., Yeates, A. J., Davidson, P. W., Shamlaye, C. F., Strain, J. J., Thurston, S. W., Harrington, D., Zareba, G., Wallace, J. M. W., & Myers, G. J. (2013). Neurodevelopmental outcomes at 5 years in children exposed prenatally to maternal dental amalgam: The Seychelles Child Development Nutrition Study. *Neurotoxicology and Teratology, 39*, 57–62.

Wolfensberger, W. P., Nirje, B., Olshansky, S., Perske, R., & Roos, P. (1972). *The principle of normalization in human services.* National Institute on Mental Retardation (Canada).

Yuan, J., Holtz, C., Smith, T., & Luo, J. (2017). Autism spectrum disorder detection from semi-structured and unstructured medical data. *EURASIP Journal of Bioinformatics and Statistical Biology, 3.* doi: 10.1186/s13637-017-0057-1.

# ABOUT THE AUTHORS

Philip W. Davidson is Professor Emeritus of Pediatrics, Environmental Medicine, and Psychiatry at the University of Rochester School of Medicine and Dentistry. He is a Pediatric Psychologist. Dr. Davidson received a BA in Psychology from Bucknell University (1963), an MS in Psychology from Villanova University (1967), and a PhD in Experimental Psychology from the George Washington University (1970). After three years of teaching and research at Washington College, Dr. Davidson completed a postdoctoral fellowship in Clinical Child Psychology at the University of North Carolina at Chapel Hill. From 1975 until 2007, Dr. Davidson directed the Department of Pediatrics' Division of Developmental and Behavioral Pediatrics and the Strong Center for Developmental Disabilities. Dr. Davidson has served as a board member or officer of number of local, state, national, and international professional and community service organizations. He served as president of the International Association for the Scientific Study of Intellectual and Developmental Disabilities (2016–19) and Division 33 of the American Psychological Association (2001–2). He is a fellow of the American Psychological Association, the International Association for the Scientific Study of Intellectual and Developmental Disabilities and the American Association for Intellectual and Developmental Disabilities. He is the 2020 recipient of the APA's Edgar A. Doll award. Dr. Davidson has over 240 peer-reviewed publications, books, and book chapters in the field of intellectual and developmental disabilities. His research focuses on the neurotoxicology of mercury, and on health and mental health of older persons with intellectual and developmental disabilities. He and his wife Margaret and their standard poodle Hercule Poirot have resided on Hilton Head Island since 2011.

Susan L. Hyman is a Professor of Pediatrics at the University of Rochester School of Medicine and Dentistry. She is Board

Certified in Pediatrics, Neurodevelopmental Disabilities, and Developmental Behavioral Pediatrics. Dr. Hyman earned her ScB in Biology from Brown University in 1976 and MD in 1979 followed by a residency in Pediatrics at North Carolina Memorial Hospital of the University of North Carolina in Chapel Hill. There, she was exposed to the interdisciplinary care of children and youth with developmental disorders. She completed at three-year fellowship in Developmental Disabilities at what was then the Kennedy Institute of Johns Hopkins Hospital and stayed on as faculty. She was the medical director of the Severe Behavior Institute there, where her research interests in Rett syndrome, challenging behavior, and autism began. After several years as a faculty member in Developmental Behavioral Pediatrics at the University of Maryland, Dr. Hyman took a clinical position at the University of Rochester in Dr. Davidson's division in 1994. Her research collaborations with Patricia Rodier, PhD, and Tristram Smith, PhD, shaped her subsequent career. Her research focus has been on diet and nutrition, medical care, and interventions for children with autism spectrum disorders. She was the chair of the Autism Subcommittee of the American Academy of Pediatrics for 14 years and spent 6 years on the executive committee of the AAP Council on Children with Disabilities. This has permitted her to advocate for the medical and behavioral needs of children and families affected by autism spectrum disorders and support their care through the medical home. These goals are further supported by her position as co-Principal Investigator of the Rochester Site of the Autism Treatment Network. She was the chair of the Sub-Board of Developmental Behavioral Pediatrics of the American Board of Pediatrics. She and her husband raised their two children and a Nova Scotia Duck Tolling Retriever in Rochester.